Lose Belly Fat

Blowout Belly Fat

Burn Fat, Lose Inches, Lose Weight and Feel Great

Belly Fat Blowout

Book 1 & Book 2

How to Burn Fat, Lose Inches, Lose Weight and Feel Great

New & Improved

Clean Eating

Healthy Eating

Fat Loss

Stephanie Atwood, M.A.

Burn Fat While Losing Inches from Your Waist, Hips and Thighs

2 Books in One!

10 Day Jump Start Plan with Details for Every Day, Every Meal

Plus Bonus Updates from Book 2

Utilize the metabolic magic that balances blood sugar, controls Type 2 Diabetes, and teach your body to burn fat, belly fat and more!

The Live Fit Series

Author Stephanie Atwood has written a number of books about health and fitness. Enclosed are photos and a link to her author page showing all her books on Amazon: http://www.amazon.com/-/e/B00BIBRX28. Leave us a review if you like what you read. Thank you again.

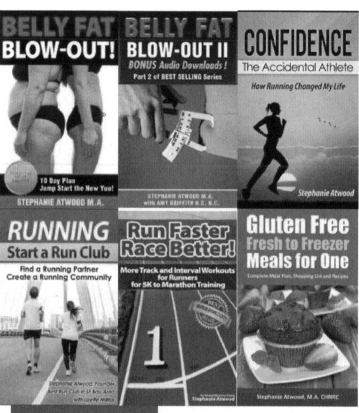

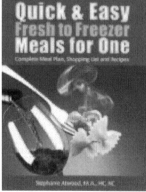

What former participants have said about the Live Fit Program:

"The program was an informative, eye opening, educational program that gave me the tools I needed to learn how to eat and workout for optimal metabolic health. Combining the expertise and experience of Running Coach Stephanie Atwood and Personal Nutrition Coach Amy Griffith created a program that was easy to follow and debunked many food myths and mysteries.

The information was presented in a clear manner along with weekly podcasts offered by Coach Stephanie & Amy. I found myself looking forward to each Friday when the newest updates and the podcasts would appear in my inbox. I loved learning how to eat the correct ratio of carbs to protein for optimum performance during my workouts and in such a way to train my body to burn fat for fuel. In addition, there is a Facebook page dedicated to the program that was a great way for all the participants and coaches to share questions, stories, recipes, victories and frustrations." – **Michaela R**

"I was originally interested in the program because I wanted to improve my running. What I found was a fantastic program that made me much more aware of just how nutrition has a huge impact on how I feel in regards to energy levels, helped me lose weight without ever feeling deprived and alleviated negative physical symptoms I was experiencing.

I liked that the program was very structured in that we got a "plan" for each week that included specific recipes rather than just general guidelines. I really enjoyed trying out the different recipes and who knew I would turn into such a fan of kale. I loved the weekly calls that summarized a lot of the *information we received via e-mail and also addressed some of the questions from Facebook. As an added bonus I could download the weekly calls to my ipod so I could listen at my convenience." – **Leti D**

Dedicated To

The eleven women who beta tested this concept for me. Without them and my program partner Amy Griffith, I would not be able to continue the series. Thanks to each of you and congratulations on your successes!

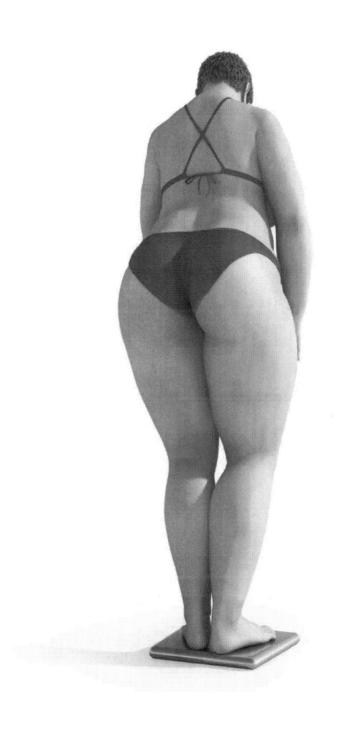

Table of Contents

The First Book

Day 10

More Recipes

Who is Stephanie Atwood, M.A?

What, Why and How

What and Why for You?

Today is the day for you to start losing your doughnut. Belly fat is not caused only by eating doughnuts. You know this and I know this. We also know that belly fat is dangerous, more so than fat thighs or hips, but too much fat anywhere is not healthy.

Would you like to know how to burn more fat?

The plan I have for you, for the next 10 days, will get you primed for burning fat. You will see a quick and positive change within the first few days, continuing throughout the 10 days of the program. Each day you will be given an exact menu to follow. The food will be delicious and you should not feel starved! Then we will transition into an eating plan that can last for the rest of your life. Sound good so far?

What is the angle?

The concept for this book was born out of metabolic efficiency training, a term I learned about through a class taught by Sunny Blende, M.S. a sports nutritionist. Metabolic Efficiency Training is the name of a book by Bob Seebohar who has written several books about nutrition and athletes. More information about Bob's books is available at the end of this book. Metabolic efficiency however, is not just for athletes. It is a way for you to train your body to utilize more fat using real food and easy exercise.

How do I know it will work?

I know it can work because I tried it first on myself and saw good results. Then I invited other women to try the program. They saw positive results, too. Their body types varied from slim to robust. Their ethnic backgrounds and ages varied as well. What did they have in common? They were willing to follow our eating plan AND were willing to walk or do some other type of exercise 6 out of 7 days a week.

I did not ask them to exercise hard or lift weights or run a marathon. I asked them to move 6 out of 7 days a week for a minimum of 30 minutes. For you, I am asking you to start with **10 minutes of walking (by Day 5)** and build from there to 30 minutes by the end of the 10 days.

Can you walk for 10 minutes and build from there? I believe you can and I KNOW you MUST be able to move for 30 minutes to have a healthy body. You know this too.

Here is what one woman says about her experience:

"This program has set me free from years of binge eating and yo-yo dieting. I have so much more energy and my sugar cravings are virtually gone. I have become passionate about healthy cooking and in making whole, real foods my "new normal." I truly believe this passion comes directly from Coach Stephanie and Amy - they are a dynamic team and have created a program that leads to success." Michaela

What?

My Story - I started the nutrition journey many years ago, right after I graduated from high school. **Why?** Well 2 major occurrences made me want to learn more about eating.

First thing: I started working as a receptionist right after graduating from high school. I was making good money for someone who had never worked a full time job before. I could afford my own apartment and wanted to leave my parents' home in a big way.

I was a receptionist and the job entailed making coffee, keeping the break room neat, and seeing that we had doughnuts every morning, in addition to my desk work. I was sitting all day, answering the phone and pushing a pencil. I ate breakfast at work which comprised one or two doughnuts and coffee with artificial creamer. I drank two or three cups of coffee before lunch. I worked. I ate lunch. I worked then went home and ate dinner. I probably had a few snacks in there too. If doughnuts were left over there is a good chance I ate another one or two at my breaks.

I gained about 25 pounds in the first 6 months of that job.

In high school we did Physical Education every day. When I started working I did nothing but sit, work, and eat all day.

Second thing: I was newly out of high school and living on my own, supporting myself! I was trying to live on a budget and figured that saltine crackers and peanut butter was a pretty cheap way to fill my belly and not spend too much money. Since I ate breakfast at work (doughnuts), I had to cover lunch and dinner. The coffee, doughnut, peanut butter and cracker menu seemed OK at the time and I was young enough that it took a while to catch up with me.

Then, all hell broke loose! I was FAT, nutritionally deficient, and totally unaware of why I felt so tired all the time.

What to do? As a young person, trying to make her own way, and enjoying my independence, I determined to start exercising to lose weight. It worked! But the way it worked was surprising...

Why?

What started out as an embarrassed, overweight, young woman hiding in the shadows of the night as she jogged around the block became an athlete who really enjoyed running, and lost weight while learning a new skill and discovering I was good at it!

As I ran faster and farther I became more interested in eating well. I could see that running used calories but, as I read and talked about running, I learned that good food would make me a better runner than eating junk food. I also learned that fresh, healthy food could be affordable. Voila! I was hooked.

The combination of losing weight with exercise and good food, while becoming a better runner, who even tried some races, convinced me that I wanted to know about both. And that is just what I did. I started a journey of more than 30 years of exploring the connection between food, exercise, and quality of life.

Now, post menopause, where many women are sporting a doughnut around their middle, I have none. My doughnut past has gone the way of my 153 pound body. NO MORE!

What I have learned is not unique. Good food, simple, healthy eating, and regular exercise has given me a better quality of life. I offer you this opportunity and give you the tools for success.

Now it is time for you to **take control and do something good for yourself**. I'm guessing that you have been thinking about this for a long time. I'm here to help! Take that first step with me. Let's get this show on the road!

How?

This starter program gets you **results FAST!**

By detoxing for 3 days you will start the process of getting your body to realize that long term change is coming. After three days we will re-introduce regular food in an eating plan that includes 3 meals and 2 snacks a day. You will not be starved and you will not be deprived of good, healthy meals. It may even surprise you that you can eat so much!

For many of the women who participated in our program, they told me they were "shocked" at how much better they felt and how the cravings disappeared. They were also a bit skeptical about how much food they could eat and not gain weight! For many of us it is the quality of the food that is changing. We may be upping the quantity because the volume is mainly in healthy, filling fruits, veggies, fats, and proteins. Yes, all of them are included in this program.

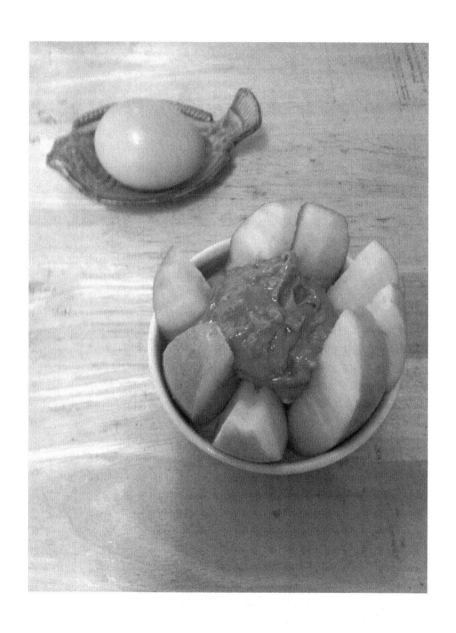

Kick Start Your New Life - Quick
Start Basics

"Today is the first day of the rest of your life".

What a wonderful opportunity we have to do good things, for ourselves and others, every day!

Ready to Kick start the NEW YOU?

All right! Let's do this!

Here are the Basics:

__ Take measurements around your waist, hips and thighs and write them here or on your calendar.

	Date	Waist	Hips	Thighs	Weight
First Day of Program – First thing in the morning					
End of 3 day Cleanse/Detox					
End of 10 days					
Keep Going!					

Plan to **start the Cleanse/Detox on a Thursday**

Start the **Get Fit program on a Monday**

Shop on Wednesday (or sooner for the Cleanse/Detox and on Sunday for the Get Fit Program so that you can shop and cook, getting ready for the work week on Monday. Your Sunday will be a free day, this first week. Thus, as you come off your detox, enjoy the day, eat without guilt (90/10 rule), shop and prepare food and get in the mind set to make your 6 week commitment starting tomorrow!

Of course you can adjust these dates to your own schedule. This is a suggested schedule and assumes that the majority of us works M-F, has kids in school those same days, etc. etc.

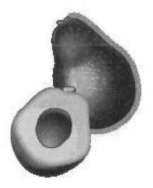

The 90/10 Rule

My health coach buddy Amy Griffith www.embracehn.com says to allow ourselves a 90/10 attitude on food. In other words, give yourself permission to "break the rules" periodically. Please don't start this on your detox program (it is, after all, only 3 days) but, in general, allow yourself the opportunity to splurge 10% of the time.

Here is the clincher. **You are the judge.** If you create a 50/50 rule and tell yourself that it's 90/10, who loses out? Be honest, practical, and fair to yourself and this program. If you follow the guidelines you will set yourself up for success. If you sabotage your own plan, you will know it.

Day 4 is a good day to try the 90/10 rule as you prepare, shop, and commit to the next 6 days of this program. 90/10 is not an exact calculation! It is giving yourself permission to eat a piece of cake at a birthday party, or an ice cream cone on a hot day. It is drinking a glass of wine or a beer once or twice a week without guilt.

If you share food with family and friends (as you can with this program); and look at physical exercise as a privilege (a gift in a body that is able to move); you are half way to success already! Now follow the day by day steps set out for you in this book and get ready to smile at how good you will feel, very soon!

10 Days of Results

As we begin this journey together I want you to trust in your judgment. Part of what you will gain from this 10 day start is an understanding of how to eat well. When you eat well you will feel good. When you feel good, you will be at peace with your body. When your body is content, because it is receiving what nutrients it needs, you will be able to lose weight, rest, control type 2 diabetes, and be less stressed. The cycle will flow.

All of us know that we are affected by stress and hormones. But we may not be nearly as clear about the layer of belly fat, around our waists, that tells us and shows us, we are stressed. This dangerous sign that sits there and frustrates us can be changed. It takes some time and it takes some re-thinking. Please hang in there. Other women have done this and you can too!

Below is your shopping list for the next three days. Please try to purchase fresh and organic when possible. If you can't find organic, don't fret. If you need to make substitutes, try to do so with your best judgment.

No kale in your supermarket? Another dark green leafy veggie is spinach or chard.

No pepitas? Raw sunflower seeds will do. DO NOT FRET!

Think, I can change things in my diet; I can learn new ways to eat; I can enjoy eating, even add to the variety of dishes for me and my family; I can eat healthy and not be burdened with an eating program that never lets me enjoy food.

You can make food a friend!

Shopping for this next 10 days is a great time to try some new things but don't fret about it. Don't spend money that you don't have but use good judgment. We want you eating as much fresh, diverse, and unprocessed food as possible without breaking the bank or stressing you in your shopping.

Three Day Detox/Cleanse

(Adapted from Get Fit with Amy Griffith H.C., N.C.
http://embracehn.com

(Check your pantry first to see if you already have some of these items before you go shopping!)

From Amy:

Get ready for a change! You are encouraged to eat unlimited veggies – and start the detox and recalibration process as you break free from the need for quick energy through sugar, caffeine and other food products that aren't serving you! Try different greens – Swiss or rainbow chard, collard greens, kale, etc. Add a variety of veggies: broccoli, red bell peppers, carrots, zucchini, kohlrabi, onions (yellow or purple), mushrooms, garlic and plenty of herbs and spices to add variety to these three days!

General Awareness – Please Read:

Please be aware of what you are eating; the quality of the food, organic produce, etc.

Refrain from processed foods, gluten (bread, pasta, white flour, crackers, chips - processed white stuff), chocolate, dairy, refined sugars, red meat, eggs, soy. **STICK WITH THE MENU!**

Water is your BEST FRIEND!

Curb sugar cravings: think of how sweet the red peppers, an apple and other fruits are in their purest form, sweet but healthful and full of fiber.

Headache? Fresh ginger in hot water might help – and keep up the water intake!

Hungry? Drink a glass of water, wait 5-10 minutes before eating more food on the menu plan.

A treat on any day can be one avocado. Feel free to eat a whole one over the course of the day (one half in the morning as snack, one half in evening, or however you want to work it).

Let's Do This!

Rather than looking at these items as too much and too many, please consider what wonderful food you will be preparing for yourself and your family and that many of the items will be available for future cooking, too.

Shopping List for the 3 Day Cleanse

Produce Checklist:

__ Arugula, big bag for green smoothies

__ Avocados, 3

__ Fruit for 3 days: bananas, (3 – 6), apples and berries for snacks and meals

__ Garlic, fresh, 1 – 2

__ Greens, various including kale, chard, spinach, bok choy, or collards. Spinach is OK raw, all the others will be used in your cooked lunches and dinners

__ Kale, 3 bunches for rice mix

__ Lemons (Meyer lemons are sweeter!), 4 – 6

__ Mushrooms, any kind, any amount

__ Onions, yellow or red, use as you like as part of your vegetable meals

__ Scallions, green onions, 9 or more

__ Various (and lots of) veggies for 3 days: red pepper, cucumber, celery, endive spears, snap peas, carrots, broccoli, cauliflower, for raw snacks, lunch and dinner

Meat/Poultry/Fish (you can alternate protein or just eat fish or chicken)

__ Roast or Baked Chicken (8 oz. legs, thighs, or breast) for 2 days

__ Wild salmon, cod or halibut, 4 oz. for 1 day

Nuts, Beans, Seeds, Grains:

__ Brown rice, 3 cups raw

__ Garbanzo beans, 2 cans

** Other beans (if not eating meat or fish): black, kidney, Navy, white northern, lentils and maybe quinoa or more brown rice to complete the protein for vegetarians)

__ Almonds, raw (no salt), 2 cups

__ Chia Seeds, 3 TBSP.... for smoothies

Condiments:

__ Tahini (sesame tahini) 1/3 cup (comes in can or jar)

__ Almond butter (raw is wonderful, chunky or smooth) small jar (usually comes in 8-16 oz.)

__ Extra virgin olive oil – to be used in almost all of your sautéing, salad dressings, and other cooking

__ Sea salt (more minerals than regular grocery store salt, colored, if possible. I've seen pink and grey)

__ Ground pepper (freshly ground makes taste more intense)

Herbs/Spices: (some or all. Use your favorites and add in a couple you haven't tried. Fresh is best, dried if needed)

__ Thyme

___ Marjoram

___ Rosemary

___ Basil

___ Parsley

___ Sage

___ Turmeric

___ Cayenne pepper

___ Paprika

___ Fresh ginger root for morning beverage and/or upset stomach

___ Green tea

___ Herb Tea

Beverages:

___ Almond milk or coconut milk (unsweetened), 1 quart for smoothies

___ Water (filtered or good, clean tap water will suffice)

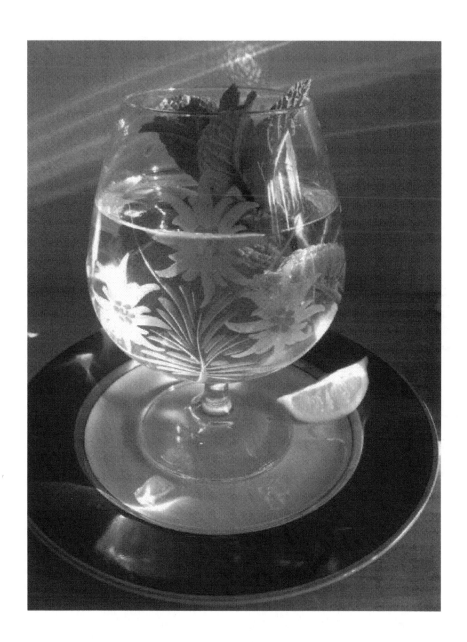

The Cleanse

Day 1-3 – Detox/Cleanse

Repeat these same foods each day. If limited for time, cook once for all three days. Eat leftovers cold, reheat prepared food, and/or make things the night before and re-blend or reheat.

Upon Rising

1. 12 oz. warm or hot water with fresh juice of one lemon or
2. Steep a few slices of fresh ginger root in boiling water, and/or
3. Green tea (in place of coffee drinks for caffeine – no sweetener) and/or
4. Any herbal tea of your choice

Breakfast (within one hour of waking)

The Green Smoothie – see recipe provided

Mid-Morning Snack (choose one of the three, not all at the same meal)

1. Any unlimited raw or steamed veggies with hummus – See Recipe, or purchase one from the store without citric acid) or
2. Handful of almonds, plain, roasted or raw, no salt or almond or peanuts butter (only containing the nuts, no sugar or other additives) with any one piece of fruit

(apples or bananas are great, or whatever is seasonal!)
or

3. ½ an avocado sprinkled with salt and pepper, plus a
   piece of any fruit

Lunch
Unlimited sautéed, roasted, or steamed greens separate or mixed
with any veggies (any color) steamed and lightly sautéed in extra
virgin olive oil or raw coconut oil (add oil towards end of cooking).
Add garlic, sea salt and pepper to taste (can also add sautéed shitake
mushrooms or onions). These can be cooked ahead of time and
eaten cold.

1/2 cup cooked brown rice (see recipe for BROWN RICE,
KALE AND SCALLIONS)

Baked or grilled chicken (skin removed) or salmon (no sauce
or marinade, only any fresh herbs, spices, or lemon juice
(salmon is great with dill, for example), salt and pepper –
light on the salt, preferably sea or Himalayan that is colored

1 half of an avocado, save half for dinner.

*Mid-Afternoon Snack: same as options for
first mid-morning snack, above, in portions
as described.*

Dinner: same as lunch but **no chicken or salmon** (only for lunch), only veggies and rice: get creative! Season with herbs and spices – fresh basil, fresh thyme, cilantro, tarragon, savory, rosemary.

Second half of avocado.

If you must have something sweet after dinner, FRUIT ONLY (one piece), a handful of berries, or try a cup of herbal tea, no sweetener.

Beverages

8-10 glasses of water throughout the day (room temperature or warm)

Herbal tea only, **no coffee, sugared drinks, wine or alcohol or dairy**

Make and sip on homemade "Mineral Broth" – a great way to fill that mineral savings account that is depleted and it's warming and delicious. I recommend Rebecca Katz Magical Mineral Broth recipe. If you can't find some of these ingredients, just leave them out:
http://rebeccakatz.com/recipes/magic_mineral_broth.html

Recipes

The Green Smoothie (Serves 1)

Best made fresh but, if needed, prepare the night before and re-blend in the morning

1 heaping handful arugula

1 spoonful almond butter (ingredients should only be almonds!)

1 banana

1 Tbsp. chia seeds

1 cup almond or coconut milk (unsweetened)

½ cup water

You can use any blender, but the more high power the blender the better! Blend on high until smooth or desired consistency has been obtained. Serve!

Spiced Paprika Hummus (Makes Approx. 3 cups)

2 (15.5-ounce) cans chickpeas, drained, rinsed

2 large cloves garlic, minced

1 teaspoon freshly squeezed lemon juice

Pinch of cayenne, paprika, or black pepper

1/3 cup extra-virgin olive oil

1/3 cup sesame tahini
Sea salt to taste

Combine the chickpeas, garlic, lemon juice, cayenne, paprika, or black pepper, olive oil, tahini and salt in a food processor or blender and process until well mixed. Add ¼ cup of water and process until smooth. Add more liquid if necessary. Scrape down the sides of the bowl once or twice. (The hummus can be made up to 3 days ahead and refrigerated). To serve, drizzle a bit of olive oil over the hummus and sprinkle a bit of paprika.

Brown Rice with Kale & Scallions (2 Servings)

Make 3 batches for 3 days for each person

1 bunch of kale (a thick, leafy green)

1 ½ Tbsp. extra virgin olive oil or raw coconut oil

2 cloves garlic, peeled & minced

3 large scallions, cut thin

2 1/2 cups cooked brown rice or quinoa
1 Tbsp. herbs of your choice

Wash and slice the kale leaves thinly. Steam the kale for 5-6 minutes. In a large saucepan over medium-low heat, heat oil. Add garlic, stir for 1-2 minutes until fragrant. Turn up heat to medium, add steamed kale and scallions. Cook for two minutes and stir in rice, cook a few minutes. Add herbs, stir, let sit for a couple minutes, then serve warm with chicken or fresh fish (halibut, salmon or cod).

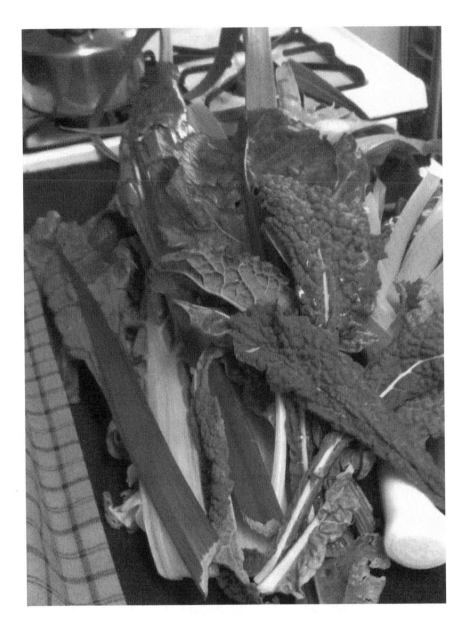

Day 4 – Relax and Prepare

Today is a day to relax both physically and mentally and get prepared for the next 6 days. You will want to shop, cook, and make that mental commitment to following through with the plan. It will take a bit of organization but it will also be fun.

If you have family who will share in this adventure, take them shopping with you! Go to the Farmer's Market if possible. You may even want to buy some seeds and start a small herb garden on your windowsill. This is a new, exciting start and can become a lifestyle as it has for some of our past participants.

You still want to **start your new day with a cup of hot water and lemon.**

Eat today in a healthy, but non restricted way. Today you will shop. Tomorrow you will be eating food that is chosen for you. Don't forget to eat breakfast, lunch, and dinner. Today is a good day to include the 90/10 rule.

You may **re-introduce caffeine. However, do not include sugar, artificial sweetener or artificial creamer, after today.** Use honey, milk (or real cream).

The next 6 days I really want you to follow the plan outlined to the best of your ability.

Remember 90/10 not 50/50 right?

Our goal for the next 6 days is to maintain a protein and carbohydrate ratio of 1:1. This means that we will attempt to balance the weight of our protein with the weight of the carbohydrates that we take into our bodies.

When you follow this eating regimen and exercise every day you are teaching your body to search for fat as fuel. Why? Because you have limited the carbohydrates and increased the protein to 50/50. You are essentially forcing your body to look for fat for energy once the store of sugar (carbohydrate) energy is depleted because fat is the second source of body energy, after carbohydrate.

We are neither limiting fat nor being excessive about it. Fat occurs naturally in many healthy types of food; meat, fish, nuts, and seeds, for example. When eating in this next 6 days you will eat fat in foods and as oil in salad dressing. We will even eat bacon!

Fat is essential to a healthy body yet, if we overeat we store the extra energy in the form of fat. The balance is to eat healthy, natural fats that come in our food but not eat too much of **Anything!** – Protein, carbohydrate or fat! This is what we are showing you in the menu provided.

Stay away from Trans Fats, hydrogenated fats such as margarine, shortening, and butter-like spreads. We encourage you to use olive oil, coconut oil, even butter. Take the skin off chicken (after cooking it) but enjoy the flavor of sautéing your food in oil, good, healthy oil. Do not deep fry food but if you are used to flavoring things with ghee or a pat of lard, this is OK in moderation, as is healthy fat, in general.

We are also **omitting ALL BREAD and Processed Flour Items such as tortillas, crackers, pasta and even cereal.** We will be staying out of the center aisles of the grocery store and staying away from most boxes of food and the frozen food aisle. We **will also avoid grains for the next 6 days**. Grains, such as oatmeal, rice, and wheat are often refined but even in their natural states, grains tend to cause inflammation and are a more complicated type of carbohydrate. By eating simple fruits and vegetables, their simple type of carbohydrate sugar will work through our bodies relatively quickly and then, voila! We will move into burning our body's fat stores for our required, additional energy for the day. Sound good? It is!

Shopping List for 6 days (some you may have already purchased or they are in your pantry. Remember to substitute when an item is not available or convenient to purchase.)

Organic and Pasture Fed when feasible

___ Applesauce, small jar, unsweetened

___ Avocados – 3

___ Bacon, 4 – 8 oz. lean, "natural" bacon, pork or turkey

___ Beef, lean cut, 6 – 12 oz. (6 oz. for each meal)

___ Celery – for snacking, lots is fine

___ Cheddar cheese – 4 oz. or small brick

___ Cherries or cranberries, dried, unsweetened – 1 cup

___ Chick peas or garbanzo beans, 1 can

___ Chicken, baked (from scratch is best, baked from store go as natural as possible) 8 – 12 oz. *(use leftovers to make soup or other meals to freeze)*

___ Coffee or Tea – 1- 2 cups a day, as you like. No artificial sweeteners but cream or milk OK

___ Cucumbers 3- 4

___ Eggs – 6

___ Feta cheese (goat or sheep)

___ Fish, fresh or frozen, non-battered, 2 pounds for filets and soup

___ Hemp Seeds, hulled, about 1 cup (these can get expensive) buy from bins in a health food store if possible. I also recommend Bob's Red Mill Brand

___ Lemons, 6 or more

___ Multi-colored peppers, 3 - 4

___ Mushrooms, lots if you like them

___ Olive Oil, cold pressed - for general use if you are purchasing new

___ Olives, Greek style or other whole olives, small jar or can

___ Onions

___ Peanut butter (no sugar added), chunky or plain, 8 – 16 oz. You may also use almond butter

___ Raw Almonds 1 – 2 cups

___ Salad Greens – mixed greens, arugula, frisee, baby kale, spinach, romaine, etc. limited iceberg for lunches and dinners

___ Sardines in oil, 1 – 2 cans

___ Spinach

___ String cheese 4 – 6, 1 oz. portions

___ Strawberries, apples, oranges, blueberries, bananas, etc. - fruit should be limited to 3 servings per day so purchase accordingly

___ Sunflower seeds, roasted and raw – 1 cup of each

__ Sweet potatoes or garnet yams, 2 small

__ Tofu, 12 oz.

__ Tomatoes, 3 – 4

__ Tuna in water, 1 – 2 cans

__ Veggies, mixed - 1 head broccoli, bok choy, Brussels sprouts, onions, carrots, fennel, asparagus, for roasting for 3 dinners (6 cups total)

__ Yogurt, Greek style, 1 quart unsweetened, non-fat, low fat or whole fat OK

Day 5

Good morning! Guess what's first on the list? Yes! Drink your hot water and lemon and savor the new day.

Today needs to **include exercise, too**. Up to this point we have just focused on food. If you have included exercise you are already ahead of the game. Movement, in the form of a noticeable effort, is an essential part of a healthy lifestyle. It doesn't need to be heavy exercise. In fact, you want to be able to talk while you move. Beware however; if you are not working up a sweat, for any of the minimum of 30 minutes you are exercising, you need to work up to that goal.

More than 30 minutes will give you more fat burning opportunity as your body needs more energy and searches for the easiest source. First it uses carbohydrates primarily then starts seeking more fat as the instant energy (from muscle glycogen [sugar]) is used up. An hour of exercise would be great because you are helping your body adapt to burning more fat by staying active longer.

Today's Exercise Goal: 10-30 minutes of brisk walking or working up to it if you aren't there yet. More is OK, too.

__ Commit to 30 minutes of exercise 6 times a week (more time is super!)

Write down the amount of time you exercised and your pulse at the end of your workout (immediately following your exercise). Use a calendar or a journal for this. Do it! Please.

Day 5 Breakfast

2 soft or hard boiled eggs

1-1oz string cheese

1 cup cooked mushrooms, onions, and spinach, or 2 cups raw celery, cucumber, multi-colored peppers

½ cup strawberries

Lemon water

Coffee or tea is OK (no artificial sweetener or creamer)

Yes, this may seem like a lot of food. You may want to eat your snack first then work into the breakfast since it would be relatively easy to cook in advance and take with you on the go. Even cook it the night before.

Snack (2 hours before lunch)

¼ cup almonds mixed with a tiny amount (open palm of hand) of (unsweetened, dried) cranberries or cherries

Drink water throughout the day

Lunch

Salad made with 4oz of cooked, chopped chicken

Greens of your choice, 2 - 4 cups total (could include spinach, endive, romaine, arugula, baby kale, cucumbers, peppers, etc.)

Scant ¼ cup sunflower seeds, salted and roasted or raw

1 small tomato

Toss all together with dressing of 1 Tbsp. Olive Oil and ½ fresh lemon, salt and pepper

Snack (2 hours before dinner)

1 Tbsp. peanut butter slathered over 2 - 4 pieces of celery or with ½ apple

½ can of tuna or sardines

Drink water throughout the day

Dinner (earlier is better than later)

6 oz. of lean beef (Substitute with 6 oz. lean chicken, pork, or fish if you don't eat beef) broiled or roasted

2 cups of roasted veggies: broccoli, onions, carrots, fennel, asparagus (a mix) cut into chunks and mixed with

½ sweet potato, scrubbed with skin left on and cut into rounds

1 Tbsp. of Olive Oil mixed with veggies, salt and pepper to taste

Roast veggies for approx. in a flat tray 15 minutes at 450 degrees, or until all veggies are tender (not cooked to death!)

Top veggies with 1 Tbsp. sprouted, salted, dried pumpkin seeds (or roast your own in a pan, briefly over medium heat).

¼ banana plus 1/2 cup of ripe blueberries or other sweet, fresh berry mixed and blended (in a blender) with ½ cup plain Greek Yogurt (no sugar added, please) and frozen while you eat your dinner. Dessert is ready!

Note: The more green veggies, the better. Carrots and yams are high on the glycemic index so a bit of moderation is called for with orange colored vegetables.

Note: We are cutting out alcohol as much as possible. Alcohol is a sugar although it is absorbed differently than other sugars. Alcohol is to be looked at as the 90/10 exception. When you drink you are consuming almost pure sugar.

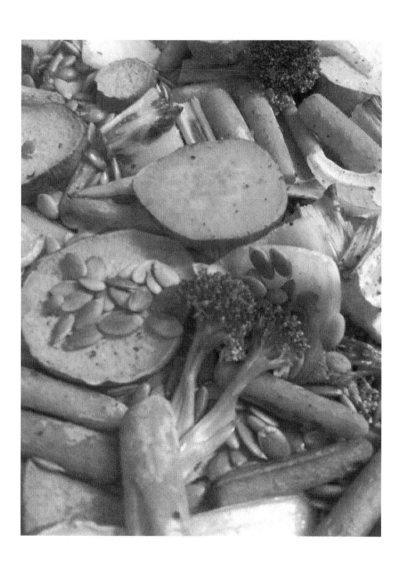

Day 6

Start with good old hot water and lemon and include a cup of coffee shortly after if it suits you.

Exercise goal for the day: 15-30 minutes of brisk walking or increasing your amount of walking by at least 5 minutes, working up to 30 minutes total. Up to 1 hour of sweating, as in boot camp would also be fine.

Breakfast

1 cup Greek yogurt (unsweetened with or without fat) mixed with

½ cup unsweetened applesauce

3 Tbsp. hulled hemp seeds or ¼ cup chopped, raw almonds or walnuts (Confirmed Ratio 1:1)

Lemon water

Coffee or tea is OK with real milk, cream, soy milk or almond milk, etc. (no artificial sweetener or creamer)

Snack

2 string cheese

1 small apple

Remember to drink water throughout the day

Lunch

½ tomato

Both hands full of mixed salad greens, dark green are best

4 Greek olives

½ deck of cards piece of feta cheese

½ cucumber

½ avocado

Salt, Pepper, 2 tsp. of olive oil and a fresh lemon squeezed on top
Mix them all together and enjoy!

Snack

½ cup hummus dip with a choice of several pieces broccoli, celery, cucumber, peppers, or asparagus

Don't forget the water!

Dinner

Lg. salad bowl, half full of salad greens (no red or orange veggies, just greens)

With ¼ cup chopped onion or scallion and ½ fresh orange slices

¼ cup roasted, salted sunflower seeds

1 lemon and up to 2 TBSP... olive oil for dressing

Pepper, no salt (it's in the sunflower seeds), all tossed together for a wonderful, refreshing, salad

½ apple and 1 oz. cheddar (or other) cheese

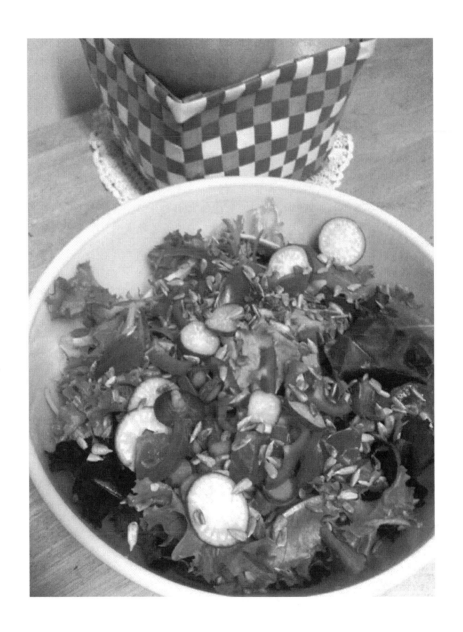

Day 7

Start with good old hot water and lemon and include a cup of coffee shortly after if it suits you.

Exercise goal for the day: 20-30 minutes of brisk walking or increasing your amount of walking by at least 5 minutes, working up to 30 minutes total. Up to 1 hour of sweating, as in boot camp would also be fine.

Breakfast

2 scrambled eggs with 2 pieces of well cooked bacon, crumbled on top or eaten on the side

Served over a bed of fresh or frozen steamed or sautéed spinach in 1 – 2 Tbsp.... Olive oil (1 -2 cups cooked), cooked with onions if time allows. *This can all be fixed the night before and reheated in the microwave if time is an issue.)*

¼ grapefruit or ½ orange (whole fruit, not juice)

Lemon water

Coffee or tea is OK with real milk, cream, soy milk or almond milk, etc. (no artificial sweetener or creamer)

Snack

¼ cup raw almonds mixed with a tiny amount of (unsweetened) cranberries or cherries

Drink water throughout the day

Lunch

Salad made with 4 oz. of cooked, chopped chicken

Greens of your choice, 2 - 4 cups total (could include spinach, endive, romaine, arugula, baby kale, cucumbers, peppers, etc.

Scant ¼ cup sunflower seeds, salted and roasted or raw

1 small tomato

Tossed with dressing of 1 Tbsp... Olive Oil and ½ fresh lemon, salt and pepper

Snack (2 hours before dinner)

A sandwich bag full of celery, cucumbers, carrots sticks, broccoli, asparagus

½ cup of satziki or hummus, yogurt and cucumber or chick pea dip

Drink water throughout the day

Dinner (earlier is better than later)

6 oz. of lean beef (Substitute with 6 oz. lean chicken, pork, or fish if you don't eat beef) broiled or roasted

2 cups of roasted veggies: broccoli, onions, carrots, fennel, Brussels sprouts, asparagus (a mix) cut into chunks and mixed with

½ sweet potato, scrubbed with skin left on and cut into rounds

1-2 Tbsp. Olive Oil mixed with veggies, salt and pepper to taste

Roast veggies for approx. 15 minutes at 450 degrees, or until all veggies are tender (not cooked to death!)

Top veggies with 1 Tbsp. roasted, salted sunflower seeds

½ ripe banana mixed and blended (in a blender) with ½ cup cottage cheese or tofu (no sugar added, please) and frozen while you eat your dinner. Add a few chopped nuts and a berry or two on top just before serving. Dessert is ready!

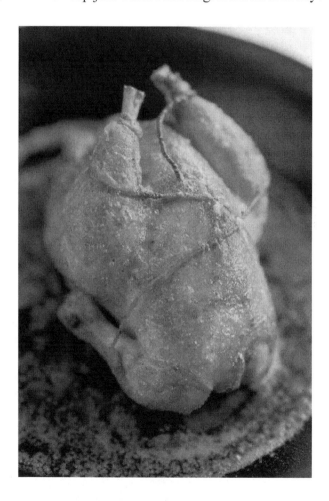

Day 8

Start with good old hot water and lemon and include a cup of coffee shortly after if it suits you.

Exercise goal for the day: 25-30 minutes of brisk walking or increasing your amount of walking by at least 5 minutes, working up to 30 minutes total. Up to 1 hour of sweating, as in boot camp would also be fine.

Breakfast

1 cup Greek yogurt (unsweetened, with or without fat) mixed with

½ banana and small handful of berries

3 TBSP. pumpkin seeds or ¼ cup chopped, raw almonds or walnuts (Confirmed Ratio 1:1)

Lemon water

Coffee or tea is OK with real milk, cream, soymilk or almond milk, etc. (no artificial sweetener or creamer)

Snack

¼ cup roasted sunflower seeds and ½ orange or ½ cup melon

Lunch

Lettuce wrap with 4 oz. of beef, turkey or tuna, 1 oz. cheese, hummus or mustard, full of salad greens. Wrap it all together like a burrito

1 small plum, peach, or apricot

Snack

1 TBSP. peanut butter slathered over 2 - 4 pieces of celery or ½ small apple

½ can of tuna or sardines

Drink water throughout the day

Dinner

Dinner

4 oz. of chicken (breast or other, skin removed) baked or broiled

Large salad bowl, half full of salad greens (no red or orange veggies, just greens)

With ¼ cup chopped onion or scallion and ½ fresh orange slices

¼ cup toasted almonds

1 lemon and up to 2 Tbsp. olive oil for dressing

Pepper, no salt (it's in the sunflower seeds)

½ apple and 1 oz. cheddar cheese

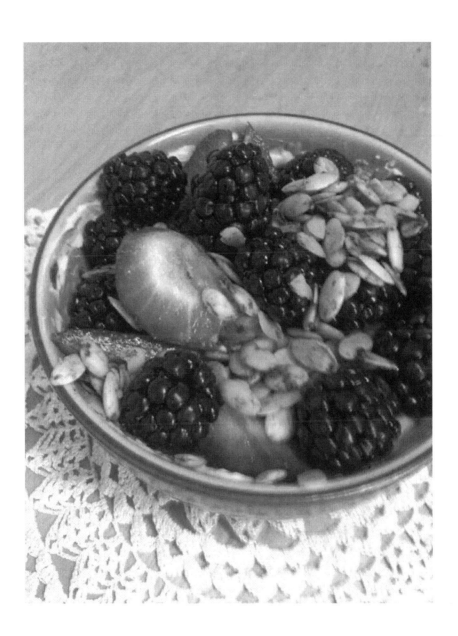

Day 9

Start with good old hot water and lemon and include a cup of coffee shortly after if it suits you.

Exercise goal for the day: 30 minutes of brisk walking. Up to 1 hour of sweating, as in boot camp would also be fine.

Breakfast

2 soft or hard boiled eggs

1-1oz. string cheese

1 cup cooked mushrooms, onions, and spinach, or 2 cups raw celery, cucumber, multi-colored peppers

½ cup strawberries

Lemon water

Coffee or tea is OK (no artificial sweetener or creamer)

Yes, this may seem like a lot of food. You may want to eat your snack, first then work into the breakfast since it would be relatively easy to cook in advance and take with you on the go. Even cook it the night before.

Snack (2 hours before lunch)

¼ cup almonds mixed with a tiny amount of (unsweetened) cranberries or cherries

Drink water throughout the day

Lunch

Salad made with 4oz. of cooked, chopped chicken or tuna (canned is OK), fresh is best

Greens of your choice, 2 - 4 cups total (could include spinach, endive, romaine, arugula, baby kale, cucumbers, peppers, etc.

Scant ¼ cup sunflower seeds, salted and roasted or raw

1 small tomato

Tossed with dressing of 1 Tbsp. Olive Oil and ½ fresh lemon, salt and pepper

Snack (2 hours before dinner)

A sandwich bag full of celery, cucumbers, carrots sticks, broccoli, asparagus

½ cup of satziki, yogurt and cucumber dip and

Nori snack pack, tasty nori snacks (once or twice a week is OK. They are high in salt but really tasty!)

Drink water throughout the day

Dinner (earlier is better than later)

6 oz. of lean beef (Substitute with 6 oz. lean chicken, pork, or fish if you don't eat beef) broiled or roasted

2 cups of roasted veggies: broccoli, onions, carrots, fennel, Brussels sprouts, asparagus (a mix) cut into chunks and mixed with

½ sweet potato, scrubbed with skin left on and cut into rounds

1-2 Tbsp. Olive Oil mixed with veggies, salt and pepper to taste

Roast veggies for approx. 15 minutes at 450 degrees, or until all veggies are tender (not cooked to death!)

Top veggies with 1 Tbsp. of roasted, salted almonds, peanuts, pepitas, or sunflower seeds

½ ripe banana mixed and blended (in a blender) with ½ cup cottage cheese or tofu (no sugar added, please) and frozen while you eat your dinner. Add a few chopped nuts on top just before serving. Dessert is ready!

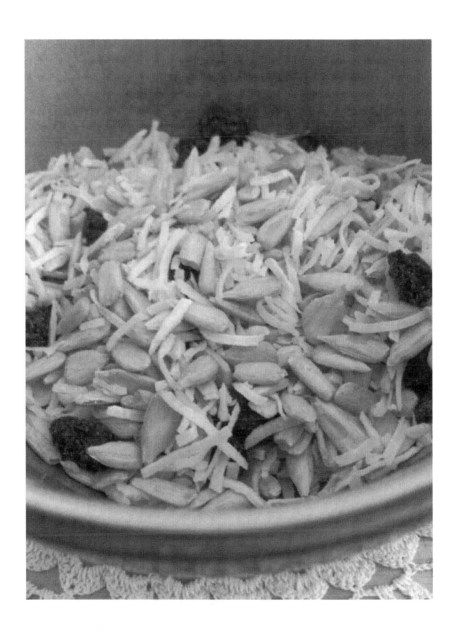

Day 10

Start with good old hot water and lemon and include a cup of coffee shortly after if it suits you.

Exercise goal for the day: 30 minutes of brisk walking. Up to 1 hour of sweating, as in boot camp or additional walking would also be fine.

Today is your day to **measure those hips, thighs, and your waist**. Write those details down on your calendar and send us a post with your results. Use our Facebook group page at http://facebook.com/getfitsuccessteam

Breakfast

Smoothie made with 1 cup unsweetened yogurt or try 1 c tofu (soft, medium, or firm)

Handful of spinach or kale

Blueberries or strawberries, ¼ cup

¼ cup applesauce

Water or almond milk to thin it. I like to add in some ice.

Cinnamon

Blend all together in a blender

Lemon water

Coffee or tea is OK with real milk, cream, soymilk or almond milk, etc. (no artificial sweetener or creamer)

Snack

¼ cup roasted or raw sunflower seeds mixed with 2 TBSP. dried, unsweetened coconut flakes and a few dry cherries, raisins, or cranberries

Lunch

Lettuce wrap with 4 oz. of turkey, ½ avocado, hummus, or mustard, full of salad greens. Wrap it all together like a burrito

1 small apple

Snack

A sandwich bag full of celery, cucumbers, carrots sticks, broccoli, asparagus

½ cup of hummus

Dinner

Seafood Chowder with bacon, fish or shell fish

Green Salad with mixed greens, no red, orange, or yellow veggies, just greens

Make enough soup to freeze some and limit the fish to 6 oz. per person when adding to the broth. Eat as much broth as you like.

½ frozen banana on a stick, just like a Popsicle

Don't forget to drink water throughout your day

Congratulations! You have finished your 10 days and now is the to time to reflect on what you have learned and how you are feeling. Even in this brief period of time you should be experiencing less cravings and burning stored fat, even that tough belly fat, along with those bulges in your hips and thighs.

Do your pants fit better? If you have been eating and exercising according to this program you will feel good, maybe even great!

Would you like to continue for another 5 weeks and see the results? Please be sure to contact us at the end of this book to join our mailing list and support group. The second book will be out shortly.

We are offering, **absolutely free,** the audio download of the first week of our Get Fit Program. Just join our mailing list and the audio download will be emailed to you, along with 2 other useful and fun handouts.

Thank you so much for making a commitment to good health through exercise and nutrition. These are key to a good life. May you be rewarded for your effort and find further resolve from your successes.

Sincerely, Stephanie Atwood

Recipes for the Rest of the 10 Days

Satziki – Cucumber Yogurt Dip (Makes 4 servings)

2 cups Greek Yogurt, non-fat, low fat or full fat is OK

1 clove garlic

2 Tbsp. olive oil

½ cucumber chopped fine

½ or whole lemon, for juice

Mix all ingredients together. Lightly salt and pepper to taste. Refrigerate for an hour or more to let flavors set as they will intensify as time goes by.

Seafood Chowder (Makes 6 servings)

6 slices bacon, cut into 1 inch pieces

1 ½ pounds of white fish, catfish, tilapia, or other white fish, cut into 6 even pieces

2 Tbsp. olive oil or coconut oil

1 chopped onion

½ cup chopped celery

½ cup chopped bell pepper, any color

½ cup chopped carrots

1 can plum tomatoes

1 cup water or chicken broth or wine

1 – 2 cups of Clamato juice or tomato juice with clam juice added for flavor

½ tsp. dry thyme or more to taste

Salt and pepper

2 or more Tbsp. chopped parsley

Sauté bacon until it is soft, about 5 minutes. Add oil and onions, celery, peppers, carrots and sauté until tender, about 10 minutes. Add the can of tomatoes, broth, juice and simmer, covered for 15 minutes. Add the fish, thyme, and salt and pepper and cook, uncovered until the fish is done, 10 – 15 minutes. Adjust the flavoring and serve with parsley on top.

This recipe may be reheated and used for more than one meal. It can be frozen also.

Optional: *Exchange chicken or turkey, or even lean sausage for the protein*

Alternate Recipe from the Author

Substitute Swiss Chard Stems for Celery

Stewed Tomatoes for Plum Tomatoes

Beer for Liquid

Skip the Clamato Juice

Add 2 cups of Swiss Chard leaves at the same time as you add the fish.

Add Italian Seasoning instead of thyme

Be creative and enjoy!

Please Leave a Review

If you were happy with the book and would like to share, I'd love to hear from you with good news. If you have suggestions for making this book better please contact me directly at go@gowowliving.com , contact us on Facebook at facebook.com/wowliving, or call 510 261-8671.

About Stephanie Atwood, M.A. and the Live Fit Program

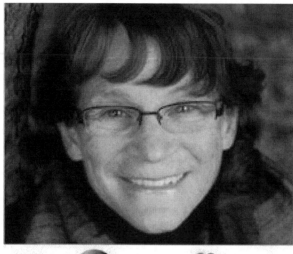

Stephanie Atwood has been writing and cooking since she was a small child. As an adult she became interested in athletics and nutrition and recently, has focused on the need for healthy, good food, for healthy, happy women by adding the nutritional component to the run and walk club that she leads Go WOW Team. http://gowowteam.com

Atwood is the Bay Area Women's Fitness Writer for examiner.com. Her articles span the breadth and depth of the Bay Area and the fascinating and diverse women in the area.

As a college educated sports nutrition consultant, health coach, and avid runner Atwood has been exploring the relationship between food and exercise and how it affects herself and the women in her club, Go WOW Team. The culmination, or possibly continuation, of that interest led to this book, the first in a series of books about eating and living well – Live Fit.

Atwood tested the fat burning, metabolic process, that utilizes exercise and food on herself before offering it to a test group of women. She lowered her own body fat from 18% to about 15%. This was tested through a lab.

She then ran a test group for 6 weeks with 11 women. The women were all willing to exercise on a regular basis but they were told NOT to exercise too hard and most of them did not consider themselves athletes. Their body types were diverse as were their ages and ethnicity.

The results were positive, informative, and educational enough that the next step seemed to be a book. This is the first in the series and now offers a sequel, Belly Fat Blowout 2.

Stephanie Atwood is also a #1 Best Selling Author on Kindle with 2 recent books on track and field.

Her dream is to bring fitness through running, walking, and good nutrition, to all ages, all body types, and all activity levels from heavy duty athletes to modest but committed active adults who are willing to move on a regular basis. Her only requirement is that people understand they are responsible to follow good, overall health practices and make small steps regularly if they are trying to change.

Thank You for Reading this Book

Congratulations!

Thank you so much for your attention to you! By this time, you are so far ahead of where you were at the beginning of your journey! Don't stop now!

If you liked this book and would like to know about new books in this Series, please join our mailing list and we will notify you of the next books in the Live Fit Series. We've included a list below of all books currently written by Stephanie Atwood:

Leave a Review

If you were happy with the book and are willing to share an honest review, we'd love to hear from you and so would other readers. If you have suggestions for making this book better please contact Stephanie directly at StephanieAwood@gowowliving.com or call 510 261-8671.

Here are the links for your review

Belly Fat Blowout 1 (go here to leave a review or purchase a copy for a friend) http://www.amazon.com/Belly-Fat-Blowout-Inches-Weight/dp/0615855024/

Other books written by Stephanie Atwood

Belly Fat Blowout 2 http://www.amazon.com/Belly-Fat-Blow-out-Management-Moderate-ebook/dp/B00D0Y7EWU/

Freezer Meals – Comfort Food
http://www.amazon.com/Freezer-Meals-Complete-Shopping-Convenience-ebook/dp/B00MRPKX58/

Freezer Meals Gluten Free
http://www.amazon.com/Freezer-Meals-Shopping-Recipes-Convenience-ebook/dp/B00N7V76OM/

Run Faster Race Better http://www.amazon.com/Run-Faster-Race-Better-Triathlons-ebook/dp/B00BPIWJP0/

Run Faster Race Even Better http://www.amazon.com/Run-Faster-Race-Even-Better-ebook/dp/B00B8BRJYA/

Journal – A Day of Achievement and Inspiration
http://www.amazon.com/Journal-Achievement-Inspiration-Stephanie-Atwood/dp/1494286149/

References and Resources

Go WOW Living - Coach Stephanie Atwood founded Go WOW Living in 2013 and Go WOW Team, the #1 Run and Walk Club in the San Francisco Bay Area. **Visit us at our website or on Facebook or Twitter** http://gowowliving.com or http://facebook.com/wowliving or @twitter.com

Contact Stephanie Atwood at go@gowowliving.com or call 510 261-8671

AtLastTheBest.com Join our VIP Club for **free (and almost free)** supplements and other products for leaving us your truthful and unbiased reviews. http://atlastthebest.com

Bob Seebohar's books about Metabolic Efficiency and Sports Nutrition. http://amzn.to/y7195c

EmbraceHN - Amy Griffith's Nutrition Website Embrace Health. http://embracehn.com

Books by Stephanie Atwood RRCA, USATF Level 2 Coach, Trainer, and Nutritionist

Author Stephanie Atwood has written a number of books about health and fitness. Here is a list with photos and a link to her author page showing all her books on Amazon.

Just click on any of the book covers to go directly to the book itself on Amazon.

Leave us a review if you like what you read. Thank you again.

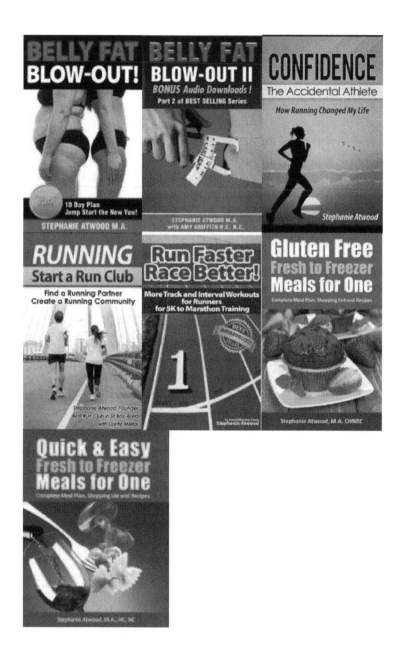

There are a few more books on Amazon, too. Take a look!

Contact Stephanie Atwood at

go@gowowliving.com

http://www.gowowliving.com

http://atlastthebest.com/

Telephone 510 261-8671

Photos in this Book

Belly Fat Blowout

Bonus Book 2

Get Fit Lose Fat

Eat Lots

Get Fit, Lose Fat, Eat Lots!

Take the Challenge!

Book 2 of the Live Fit Series

Are you ready to:

Burn Fat

Lose Inches

Boost Metabolism

Balance Blood Sugar

Control Type 2 Diabetes

Eat Real Food without Guilt

And more

Continue what you started in Book 1

First in the Best Selling Live Fit Series

Here is what readers are saying about

Book #1, Belly Fat Blowout

"The author gives you a step-by-step plan for losing belly fat fast." **Jennifer Silva**

"It's step-by-step and easy to follow." **John S. Rhodes**

"I can't wait to get started on this 10 day jump start plan!" **Kristy B.**

"As someone who has struggled for YEARS with sugar addiction, I welcomed the challenge to learn how to eat in such a way that I a) Did not feel deprived and b) Could kick the "sugar monster" out for good. Atwood presents the material in a very easy to understand manner and suddenly things just click....Not just another "diet" book - but a way to change your way of thinking about food and in turn a way to move toward a more healthy lifestyle." – **Michaela R.**

If you would like to **see more reviews,** follow this link
http://amzn.to/ZkB8A2

From a Former Participant in the Get Fit Program

"I was originally interested in the Get Fit program because I wanted to improve my running. What I found was a fantastic program that made me much more aware of just how nutrition has a huge impact on how I feel in regards to energy levels, helped me lose weight without ever feeling deprived and alleviated negative physical symptoms I was experiencing.

*I liked that the program was very structured in that we got a "plan" for each week that included specific recipes rather than just general guidelines. I really enjoyed trying out the different recipes and who knew I would turn into such a fan of kale. I loved the weekly calls that summarized a lot of the information we received via e-mail and also addressed some of the questions from Facebook. As an added bonus I could download the weekly calls to my iPod so I could listen at my convenience." – **Leti D**

Are you ready to launch your new life?

Copyright Page

Disclaimer

This book is designed to provide helpful information on the subjects discussed. This book is not meant to be used, nor should it be used, to diagnose or treat any medical condition. For diagnosis or treatment of any medical problem, consult your own physician. The publisher and author are not responsible for any specific health or allergy needs that may require medical supervision and are not liable for any damages or negative consequences from any treatment, action, application or preparation, to any person reading or following the information in this book. References are provided for informational purposes only and do not constitute endorsement of any websites or other sources. Readers should be aware that the websites listed in this book may change.

This book is designed to provide information and motivation to readers. It is sold with the understanding that the publisher is not engaged to render any type of psychological, legal, or any other kind of professional advice. The content of any article is the sole expression and opinion of its author, and not necessarily that of the publisher. No warranties or guarantees are expressed or implied by the publisher's choice to include any of the content in this volume. Neither the publisher nor the individual author(s) shall be liable for any physical, psychological, emotional, financial, or commercial damages, including, but not limited to, special, incidental, consequential or other damages. Our views and rights are the same: You are responsible for your own choices, actions, and results.

Dedicated To:

The teachers who taught me about nutrition; the family that taught me to love food; the mentors who shared their skills in the outdoors; without all of them I would not be where I am now, asking questions, getting answers, loving food and grateful every day for the gift of movement!

- Stephanie Atwood

Thank you to my family who always challenge me, to my friends who try out my recipes and support my experiments, to Bauman College staff and their tireless dedication to whole foods nutrition, and to my incredible husband for his support, patience and unconditional love for me and my passion: helping others find food again.

- Amy Griffith

Table of Contents for Belly Fat 2

Chapter 1

Belly Fat Blowout Book 1 - A Review

Welcome to Belly Fat Blowout and the Get Fit, Lose Fat, Eat Lots Program. The outpouring of positive feedback to the first book in this series, Belly Fat Blowout, has been incredible!

People, like you, are reaping the benefits of this innovative concept and the results it creates. This makes me very proud and pleased.

This second book, Belly Fat Blowout II, is a 5 week continuation of the program started in Book 1. By the time you complete Book 2 you will have established eating and exercise patterns that can guide you through the rest of your life. New habits will have time to form and solidify.

You have already completed the basics from Book 1 which took you through the pre-program cleanse and detox. I then introduced you to the foundation of eating at a protein/carbohydrate ratio of 1:1 and exercise at a minimum of 30 minutes, 6 times a week.

Now that you know the basics, we will give you more information and more food ideas.

As long as you include 30 minutes of movement, 6 times a week (more is fine); you will fill the movement component.

Please note that this concept works for athletes as well as non-athletes. Book 4, in the series, will take you through eating and training with an athlete in mind.

You are READY to take the challenge but **are you WILLING** to take the challenge?

Does having more energy, losing inches, creating a strong heart, and controlling things like blood sugar and type 2 diabetes, sound like a good way to live your life? Does enjoying food with others sound like a good way to make life more pleasant? Does eating meals with your family sound like a goal worth moving toward? Does sharing an active excursion with friends or family, that all can participate in, appeal to you?

These are goals to strive for with this program. Amy and I want you to **get fit, lose fat, and be able to eat good, quality, Real Food!** Lots of it!

Your mission, should you decide to accept, is to face this challenge with an open mind, a willing body, and an understanding that Amy and I believe in you! When **You believe in You**, half of the challenge is over. The second half is to stick with the plan. The details are described below.

You can do it!

Stephanie Atwood, M.A.

Best Selling Author and Coach

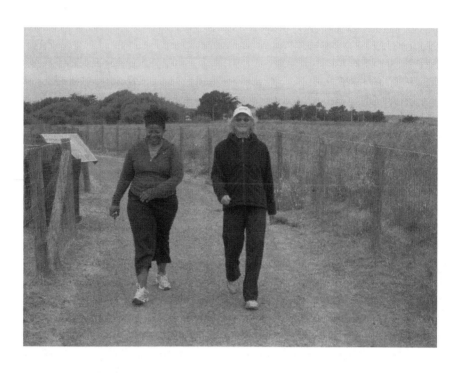

Walking is such a great form of exercise!

Chapter 2

Details

Welcome to Get Fit, Lose Fat, Eat Lots! A program developed by Amy Griffith and me. Get Fit takes Belly Fat Blowout, Book 1, and moves it up a notch, into a lifestyle.

I want to introduce my co-author Amy Griffith, certified Health Coach and Nutrition Consultant, who brings a wealth of knowledge, enthusiasm, and inspiration to the mix. Amy is a terrific example of living what she believes in. She has taken the time to learn her trade from the Institute of Integrative Nutrition and Bauman College.

Amy and I worked together with our first "in house" group of participants in Get Fit, and both of us benefitted from the synergy. You will too. I wrote Belly Fat Blowout Book 1 as a result of my own experience and the group's experience using the Get Fit Concept.

Get Fit, Lose Fat, Eat Lots

Movement and Whole Foods Create Good Health

Program Details from Book 1

If you haven't already read Belly Fat Blowout, Book 1, we highly recommend reading and following Book 1, before starting this book. Your first 10 days of this program come from that book.

In Book 1 we started off with a 3 day cleanse/detox to introduce your body to a new phase. After following the cleanse we took you through 7 days of the Get Fit Program. That is Week 1 in this book.

The remaining 5 weeks, covered in this book, and supported with audio downloads for each week, will give you the opportunity to learn, practice, and think of this new way of eating as a lifestyle, not a diet, not a quick fix, but a way of living well.

This is the Get Fit Challenge!

You too can feel better, lose inches, and have more energy. Here is a **recap of Week 1**, after the cleanse.

1. We gave you a shopping list to support the recipes and meal suggestions that were included. You can refer back to those recipes and meal ideas at any time during the next 5 weeks. Of course, there will be more in this book but we highly recommend starting at the beginning with the first book.

2. We talked about exercise/movement. By now, you are up to 30 minutes or more of sweat inducing movement 6 days a week. Our #1 recommended movement is walking because this works for almost every age and ability. The caveat with walking is that you need to work up a sweat!

3. 1:1 Ratio of protein and carbohydrate (in the form of fruits and vegetables) is our goal for the next 5 weeks. You can always fall back on the meals in Book 1 because they are set to a 1:1 ratio if you become confused or just want something simple. The 1:1 ratio utilizing lean protein and fruits and vegetables (no grains or processed foods of any kind) is essential to success.

4. We are avoiding grains and processed foods. This may be the toughest one to understand and adjust to because almost all of us base our eating around bread, rice, and/or potatoes! From Book 1, you have already been doing this if you are following the menu.

5. Moderation in Portions, Ratio of 1:1. We all know what makes a reasonable portion for our needs. Unfortunately we often revert to other rationale to tell us how much we need. But, in truth, **we know!** We are not counting calories in this program but, if you eat a jar of peanut butter for lunch, is that a reasonable portion?

6. **Start with Protein** for balancing 1:1. When you are choosing how much to eat, start with a **reasonable sized portion of protein** then add an equal amount of carbohydrate, based on density (weight). So, a 4 - 6oz piece of fish should be accompanied with 4 - 6 oz. of vegetables.

7. **The 90/10 Rule**. Allow a 90/10 approach to food. Give yourself permission to "break the rules" periodically. In general, allow yourself the opportunity to splurge 10% of the time, stay with the plan 90% of the time.

90/10 is not an exact calculation! It is giving yourself permission to eat a piece of cake at a birthday party, or an ice cream cone on a hot day. It is drinking a glass of wine, a small soda, or a beer once or twice a week without guilt.

Remember the clincher. You are the judge. If you create a 50/50 rule and tell yourself that it's 90/10, who loses out? Be honest, practical, and fair to yourself and this program. If you follow the guidelines you will set yourself up for success. If you sabotage your own plan, you will know it.

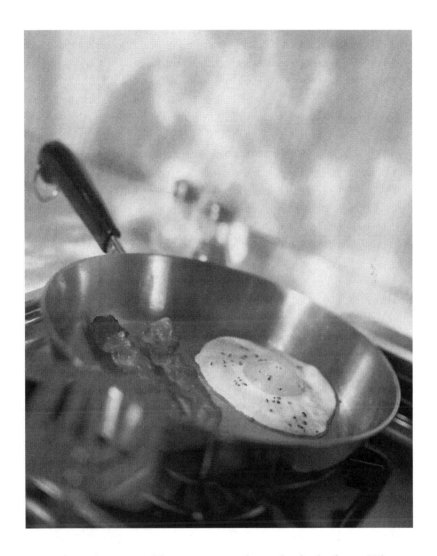

Bacon and eggs! Add some avocado and a little fruit. What a great breakfast.

Chapter 3

Moving Ahead

Why does Get Fit, Lose Fat, Eat Lots work? It has to do with kick starting your body to burn fat. Many processed foods (including bread, crackers, muffins, etc.) create a blood sugar spike because of the processed flour and sugar in almost all of them. When this happens, your body will use that "instant energy" if it needs a boost and, if not, it will have to store that energy as fat. We want your body to USE fat, not STORE fat.

We are trying to kick start a process, by eating fruits and vegetables as your only carbohydrate AND exercising to use up the immediate stores of sugar in your blood. When that instant energy is gone, you are FORCING your body to hunt for FAT to help keep you going. Fat is the second source of energy for your body.

Why no grains? Grains are carbohydrates as are fruits and vegetables BUT they are more complex molecules and therefore, take longer to digest. Omitting grains entirely is what you started in Week 1 from Book 1. Just keep it going another 5 Weeks and then you can let up a bit – Promise!

Even skinny looking people have plenty of fat stored in their bodies but, to get access to that energy, you first need to use the immediate stores of sugar energy (carbohydrates) in your blood. Then, when it's not so easy to just reach out and grab for the sugar, your body will resort to burning fat.

Thus, if you exercise at a steady pace for 30 minutes (an hour is better), don't eat during that time, and start from a meal that was 1:1, you will likely push the meter toward fat burning. I have tried it myself and saw the results. I have worked with others and they, too, saw results.

Here is what happened:

Lost fat, **increased lean body mass**

Lost weight **from actual fat, not muscle**

Lost inches, **in waist, hips, and thighs**

Lost cravings **for sweets**

P.S. After 6 weeks you can add grains back in. You'll know better how to coordinate and mix to allow for the whole grains balance so you don't undo your successes up to that point!

P.P.S. For 6 weeks we're asking you to stay away from all foods made with flour (bread*, cakes, cookies, tortillas*, crackers) and/or processed foods. There is one type of tortilla and one type of bread we have found that are flourless!

*Please look on the label and if it is **ENTIRELY Sprouted Grains with NO Flour, it is a GO!** Some great brands we know of are Ezekiel, Alvarado Street and French Meadow Bakery.*

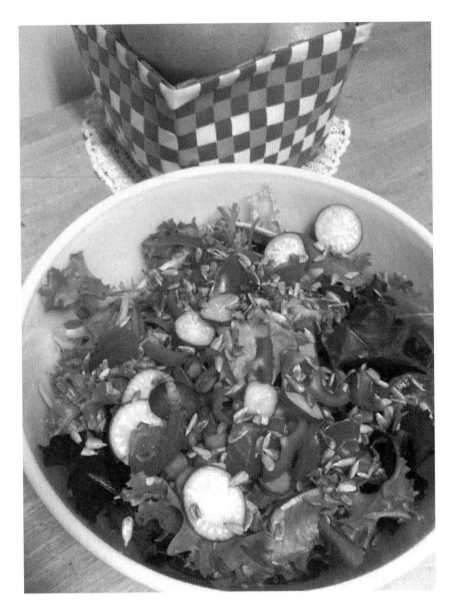

Big bowl of salad. Mixed leafy greens and other colors of veggies.

Chapter 4

New Stuff

We are now entering new material for your successful completion of this fat burning program. This program works for all kinds of people who would like to burn more of their stored body fat. Who wouldn't?

Each week's support call is available to you for download, to listen to and learn from at your convenience. Those calls are listed at the end of each week's chapter.

We are adding additional meal plans in this book. The ratio, however, needs to become a concept that you can use for many meals. Once you understand the basics and practice through actual eating, you will get a sense of what a 1:1 ratio feels like and will not need to measure or be limited to just a few foods.

Where's the Fat? Using this 1:1 ratio excludes "counting" fat. Why? When you eat healthy protein and fruits and vegetables, there is fat in the food. Healthy fats (like those in seeds, nuts, and lean protein) are essential to a functional, fit body. Other fats and oils will be used in small amounts for salad dressing or cooking but will be unrefined and unprocessed whenever possible. For example, we've included salad dressing recipes to replace store-bought varieties.

We recommend trying the following test to get a healthy visual image of what 1:1 looks like when using real food.

First, weigh out a moderate portion of fish or chicken on a food scale (one with grams and ounces is great). For most of us that would be 4 – 6 oz. for a meal. Then, take a bag of mixed greens (salad mix of some type) use a plastic bag and start filling the bag on the scale until it reaches the same amount of weight, 4 – 6 oz.

When we tried this eyes popped out of our heads! WOW! That is a lot of green stuff. While most of us might not eat such a large salad, by adding other colors and types of vegetables (carrots, cabbage, cucumbers, onions, radishes, kale, etc.) you will make a more interesting (and dense) mix that will create an equal ratio of protein to carbohydrate but doesn't take a huge mixing bowl to hold your portion!

Or, you could eat a smaller salad and add another vegetable on the side. Green is best. Add asparagus, broccoli, spinach, etc. What about some avocado or a couple of olives? Yes, they are vegetables, too.

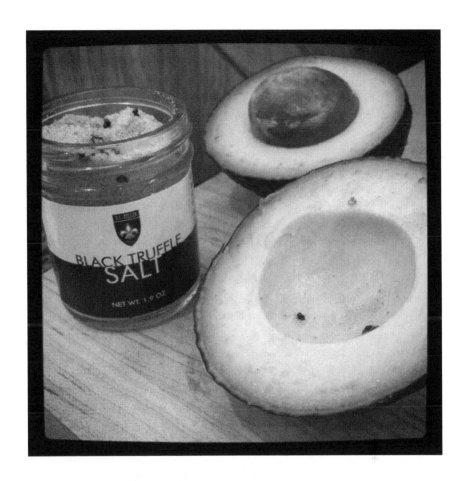

Half now, half later. What a treat!

Chapter 5

In More Depth

You will receive additional recipes and handouts each week. Check at the end of Chapter 6, in the Resources Section, for the materials available to you for this first week.

Each week includes an additional recorded call. Some of you may have already received Call #1. It was offered as a free download when you joined our Get Fit Interest List. It is also listed at the end of Chapter 6.

Sweat

I have seen many women set out to "exercise" and never work up a sweat. When I ask them to take their pulse, it is not high enough to make their hearts work hard enough to get stronger.

You MUST walk or do some form of exercise that raises your heart rate if you want to stay fit. While good intentions and any movement are laudable, to burn fat and improve your overall fitness you MUST make enough **effort to raise your heart rate**. I have written a detailed explanation of sweating and your heart rate and attached it **in the Resources Section.**

I have heard that some people do not sweat so if this is YOU, please learn to take your pulse and keep it at approximately 65% of your MHR (Maximum Heart Rate). This method is also useful to check against your level of effort, even if you do work up a sweat. It can confirm the results and let you know you're not working too HARD!

The goal is to work between 65 – 70% and, in general, is based on age. The formula you can use is listed at the end of Chapter 6 under Resources.

1:1 Ratio – Carbohydrate to Protein - Reading Food Labels

In addition to getting a sense of proportion for carbohydrate to protein by weighing out things and by using the foods that you ate during your first week (which were measured out for you) we will teach you about reading food labels. Food labels are, most often, on processed foods. When you take a look at them it can be quite an eye opener.

For example, I bought some Kashi Go Lean Crunch, a relatively healthy cereal, as cereals go. I looked at the Nutrition Facts on the back. Here is what it told me, in brief:

Nutrition Facts

Serving Size 1 Cup (53g/1.9 oz.)
Servings Per Container About 27

Amount Per Serving

Calories 190   Calories from Fat 25

	% Daily Value*
Total Fat 3g	5%
Saturated Fat 0g	0%
Trans Fat 0g	
Cholesterol 0mg	0%
Sodium 100mg	4%
Potassium 300mg	9%
Total Carbohydrate 37g	12%
Dietary Fiber 8g	32%
Soluble Fiber 3g	
Insoluble Fiber 5g	
Sugars 13g	
Protein 9g	14%

Vitamin A 0%	•	Vitamin C 0%
Calcium 4%	•	Iron 10%
Phosphorus 10%	•	Magnesium 10%

Ingredients: Kashi Seven Whole Grains and Sesame Blend (whole: Hard red wheat , brown rice, barley, triticale, oats, rye, buckwheat, sesame seeds)soy protein concentrate, evaporated cane juice crystals, brown rice syrup, chicory root fiber, whole grain oats, expeller pressed canola oil, honey, salt, cinnamon, mixed tocopherols (natural Vitamin E) for freshness.

Serving Size 1 Cup (53g/1.9oz.)

We will spend more time looking at labels throughout the course. Today I would like you to look at the Carbohydrate and Protein Ratio from Kashi. 37:9 comes from 37 grams of carbohydrate to 9 grams of protein in a serving of 1 cup. If we do simple math and divide 37/9 we will come out with approximately 4:1 (There are 4 parts of carbohydrate in one serving of cereal for each part of protein.

What does this tell us? In a simple way, this tells us we need to add more protein to get our ratio back to 1:1.

What do we add? A piece of lean bacon and an egg is adding almost all protein.

1/2 cup of milk on the cereal is about 1:2 Carbohydrate to Protein so you are adding more protein than carb to the mix.

In general we recommend keeping your carbohydrates and protein ingredients as "clean" as possible. Meaning, mix pure protein with pure carbohydrate. This not difficult when you stick with whole foods. It becomes quite difficult when you start adding in packaged, processed stuff. Then you get in trouble. Stay away from the packages and you will be a much happier camper, guaranteed.

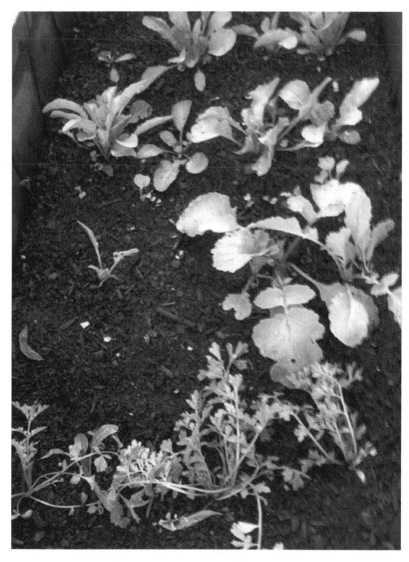

Shop the perimeter of the store! Better yet, start a garden!

Chapter 6

What Else?

The First Week's Call

As you know, you have access to a support call with each new week. Some of you may have already listened to this call. It might be worth listening to again! Amy and I want to commend you for taking this journey with us. Here is a brief review of what you can expect in that first call.

a) Encouragement to stick with the plan
b) Food Ratio Talk
c) Water, why water?
d) Fat, yes we want you to eat fat and we'll tell you why
e) Diet Soda, unfortunately a no-no. Time to start breaking the habit. Amy tells you why and offers some options.

Food Journal

Maybe you already started a food journal. If not, we suggest that you do so TODAY! You can make your own version or, if you wish, use the suggested journal I found on Amazon. Here is the link http://amzn.to/ZhmH3B. A great way to share this information with us is via the Facebook page at http://Facebook.com/GetFitSuccessTeam. We will comment on whatever you send and will NEVER be critical, only supportive.

New Recipes

Access them at the end of this section.

Feeling Hungry? Confused? Please post questions and comments on Facebook

General Reminders:

This is not a diet, per se; it is a way of life that includes movement and eating as part of a whole life system. It is a fitness and eating plan, for a healthy lifestyle, that offers weight loss and fat burning as additional benefits. When you eat well and add movement to the mix, cravings go away and you feel better! Your clothes will also fit better because swelling and actual lumps and bumps of fat can go away.

Carbohydrate - Fruit ok, unlimited veggies

Grains – Omit for first 6 weeks total. This includes all flour products (bread, etc.) but also includes rice, quinoa, pasta, barley, potatoes, etc. If you have followed Book 1, that was already your first week, and you have 5 more weeks of omitting grains entirely.

Protein – Always with a meal! **With every meal**

Fats – healthy fats, reasonable portion of these whole foods – refer to your good vs. bad fats handout to see what fats are best – a HANDFUL of any food, 1-2 tbsp. of oil per meal

Women who have been on yo-yo diets for a long time: just as much as it takes a decade or more to gain 2-3 pounds here and there a year, and all of a sudden you are in trouble – it takes a while to re-train your brain out of bad habits and inherit good ones, so be patient, don't give in to "bad days". We want to get you to a WEIGHT EQUILIBIRUM. It is hard to "just lose weight already!" as some of you may have heard before, over and over. We understand and are here to support you in this journey.

Just as much as Stephanie can't run for you, we can't eat for you – but we are here for you, to support you, cry and laugh with you if you need it, as much as you need. Take advantage of us! Contact us on Facebook.

Keep in mind the weight of the protein portion vs. the amount of vegetables to equal it for reasonable portions.

*We call the program **Get Fit, Lose Fat, Eat Lots** because, as long as you act reasonably, you can eat real amounts of real food. No artificial, non-fat, tasteless, non-food items here! Your guideline is common sense and a food plan that will fill your nutritional needs along with a movement plan that will keep your physical body healthy.*

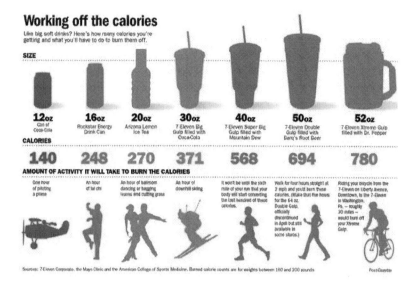

Working off the calories

Like big soft drinks? Here's how many calories you're getting and what you'll have to do to burn them off.

SIZE

12oz	16oz	20oz	30oz	40oz	50oz	52oz
Can of Coca-Cola	Rockstar Energy Drink Can	Arizona Lemon Ice Tea	7-Eleven Big Gulp filled with Coca-Cola	7-Eleven Super Big Gulp filled with Mountain Dew	7-Eleven Double Gulp filled with Barq's Root Beer	7-Eleven Xtreme Gulp filled with Dr. Pepper

CALORIES

| 140 | 248 | 270 | 371 | 568 | 694 | 780 |

AMOUNT OF ACTIVITY IT WILL TAKE TO BURN THE CALORIES

| One hour of piloting a plane | An hour of tai chi | An hour of ballroom dancing or bagging leaves and cutting grass | An hour of downhill skiing | It won't be until the sixth mile of your run that your body will start consuming the last hundred of these calories. | Walk for four hours straight at 2 mph and you'd burn these calories. (Make that five hours for the 64 oz. Double Gulp, officially discontinued in April but still available in some stores.) | Riding your bicycle from the 7-Eleven on Liberty Avenue, Downtown, to the 7-Eleven in Washington, Pa. — roughly 30 miles — would burn off your Xtreme Gulp. |

Sources: 7-Eleven Corporate, the Mayo Clinic and the American College of Sports Medicine. Burned calorie counts are for weights between 160 and 200 pounds.

Post-Gazette

At 100 calories per mile of walking, how long do you have to walk just to even out the calories consumed in a 52 oz. soft drink?

Handouts, etc. from Week 1

If links are very long, sometimes it is better to copy them into your address bar because, by default, they may end up getting cut off before the entire link is read *(if it is not on one continuous line).*

Get Fit Cheat Sheet
http://www.mediafire.com/file/cffysesygd3f5f2/GET_FIT_Cheat_Sheet.docx

Good Fat Bad Fat
http://www.mediafire.com/file/wcfflz2eka78a1c/Good_vs_Bad_Fats_handout.pdf

Morning Mantras
http://www.mediafire.com/file/94k8qfv393dwe19/Embrace_Health_Mantras.pdf

Your Ideal Day Timeline
http://www.mediafire.com/file/x4medodq5wdxa8p/GET_FIT_Your_Ideal_Day_timeline.pdf

Recipes and Meal Options #1
http://www.mediafire.com/file/0ck7wk1mvml9e3a/GET_FIT_Meal_Plan_WEEK_1.pdf

Sweat and Pulse/Heart Rate Information
http://www.mediafire.com/file/99m4j0nkaz2u8p0/Measuring_Sweat_and_Pulse_for_Healthy_Movement.pdf

Week 1 Resources and Reference Material

Facebook http://Facebook.com/GetFitSuccessTeam

A Food Journal http://amzn.to/ZhmH3B

Audio – use our calls as a resource to listen to any time

MP3 Version:

http://www.mediafire.com/file/pp513bn1n1v8hx7/Get_Fit,_Lose_Fat,_Eat_Lots_Week_1.mp3

On to Week 2!

Nutrition Facts

Serving Size (30g) 1.1 OZ
Servings per container: 15

Amount Per Serving

Calories 110   Calories from fat 25

% Daily Value*

Total Fat 2.5g	4%
Saturated Fat 0g	0%
Trans Fat 0g	
Cholesterol 0mg	0%
Sodium 0mg	0%
Total Carbohydrate 20g	7%
Dietary Fiber 2g	8%
Sugars 9g	
Protein 3g	

Vitamin A 0%   Vitamin C 0%   Calcium 2%   Iron 6%

* Percent Daily Values are based on a 2000 calorie diet. Your daily values may be higher or lower depending on your calorie needs.

Calories:		2,000	2,500
Total Fat	Less than	65g	80g
Saturated Fat	Less than	20g	25g
Cholesterol	Less than	300mg	300mg
Sodium	Less than	2,400mg	2,400mg
Total Carbohydrate		300g	375g
Dietary Fiber		25g	30g

Calories per gram:
Fat 9 • Carbohydrate 4 • Protein 4

INGREDIENTS: 100% whole grain rolled oats, almonds, honey, molasses, craisins (cranberries, sugar), raisins, sunflower seeds, cinnamon.

100% PURE & NATURAL WHOLE GRAIN GRANOLA
NOTHING ARTIFICIAL.
NO PRESERVATIVES.
NATURAL ANTIOXIDANTS.

Contains gluten and tree nut.
Manufactured in a facility that also uses wheat, soy, and dairy.

0 47097 00010 0

The 20g of carbohydrate in this granola creates a ratio of approx. 6:1 carbs to protein. This is not a good food to use for the first 6 weeks unless you add a large additional amount of protein to it. If this granola has 20g in a normal portion you'll need approx. 17 grams of protein. Two eggs or ½ cup cottage cheese would accomplish this.

Chapter 7 Week 2

Moving Forward

Thanks for getting engaged in the program! We admire your dedication and interest in your health. As you know, you will be receiving additional recipes, handouts, resources and links to a new call, every week, to enliven your experience.

As we start Week 2 here are a few things to check off once per week. We recommend starting each week on Sunday so that you can shop, cook, and plan for the next 7 days.

The Checklist

___ Measure **your hips, thighs and waist** with a tape measure. Try on that pair of slacks that is a bit too tight and check it each week. Your clothes will loosen up in your "fat storing" areas as you follow the program. Go for it!

___ **Take a photo of yourself**, full body, dressed in form fitting workout clothes. We ask you to do this at the start of each week and post your photo where it will remind you of your goal – **fat burning, life balancing, making a commitment and sticking with it.**

___ **Check your calendar** to confirm that you have 6 days of movement scheduled.

___ **Shop and prepare** a meal plan for the next 7 days. You have help from us with menu ideas in the Resource Section at the end of each week.

___ Whether you write this down or make a mental note please consider these aspects of your eating:

1. **Nutrition:** Time of day (length of meal), Food (amount and type), Where and with Whom? Feelings, before and after meal

2. **Supplements**: Amount and time taken

3. **Activity and Exercise:** Time started (energy level/emotions), Type of Activity, Length of time (heart rate at end of exercise), Where?

A Review of Last Week's Information

Last week we went over the 1:1 carb to protein ratio concept, good vs. bad fats, water and proper hydration, diet soda, sweat and heart rate. We encouraged you to fill out a food journal and give us feedback on Facebook.

There is no stupid question and our comments will be nothing but supportive – we've got your back!

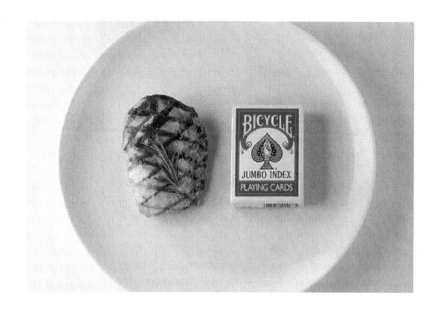

A reasonable portion of
cooked chicken. About 6 oz.

Topics Covered on This Week's Call

We discuss the importance of fiber; what it is and the different types.

1) Women should be getting 25 grams, men 38 grams (according to the Institute of Medicine). The average American gets 10 grams per day but should be getting 14 grams of fiber for every 1,000 calories.

We add details to why no grain and processed foods.

1) Grain is a more complex carbohydrate and takes longer to get through your system. Thus, it slows down the process of using fat for energy because the body will choose carbohydrate first, if it is in your system, before burning fat.

2) Processed food, including all flour products raises the blood sugar level.

We review your exercise needs and go over low intensity details. Why and How?

Amy and I discuss electrolytes in detail; when to drink; why we advocate certain drinks like coconut water and even home-made energy drinks; why we don't recommend Gatorade or many of the synthetic, non-sugar electrolyte drinks, and we give you some alternatives, such as:

1) Natural electrolyte drinks like coconut water and chocolate milk.

2) Home-made version - add mineral salt to your coconut water or make your own warm water with lemon and tsp. sea salt or grey salt with the natural minerals and without the sugar

2) Synthetic drinks without sugar like Nuun, vitamin drinks, and others

3) Synthetic drinks with sugar like Gatorade, Cytomax, Accellerade, etc. (high fructose corn syrup in the store bottled drinks)

4) Other forms of electrolytes like capsules, drops, etc.

We talk about snacks, what and when to eat for exercise.

A Bit More

Good health and fitness come from a melding of nutrition, exercise, and joy in living overall. We recommend reading Michael Pollan's Book (link in Resources), *In Defense of Food*. It offers an education and healthy approach to food, eating, and living well.

As important as it is to eat healthfully throughout this process, remember your exercise goals, low intensity requirements, and making time to rest, recover and relax. Get a massage, try out a yoga class or meditate. Find time to enjoy some peace and quiet daily.

Try a new food out this week and report back to us via Facebook – have fun with it!

That's it for Week 2. Be sure to look over the Handouts and Resources. You are making great progress!

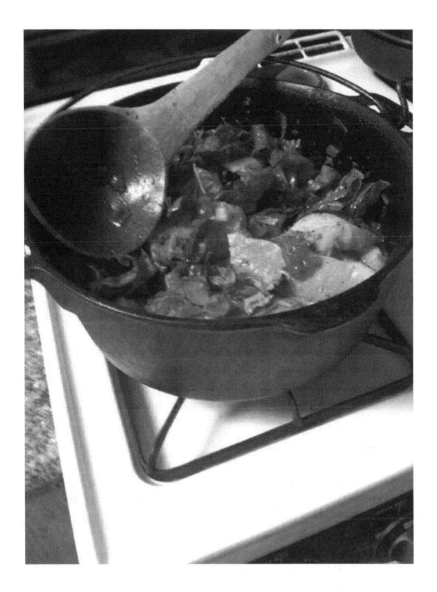

Home-made soup. Make a big batch and freeze some!

Some Questions

1. How is the exercise going? Are you measuring your heart rate?

2. Are you using Facebook as a resource? If yes, tell us what you think about it. If not, why?

3. What is your favorite way of making water more exciting?

4. How did your food journal help you to be more mindful around what foods you were eating?

Handouts, etc. from Week 2

Weekly Food Prep Routine
http://www.mediafire.com/file/wry1t3muy5tkh1m/Weekly_Food_Prep_Routines.pdf

Recipes and Menu Options #2
http://www.mediafire.com/file/uzon9o32woeyntl/Get_Fit_Week_2_Menu_Options.pdf

Water!

http://www.mediafire.com/file/srgnvzt2lzr18zd/WATER.pdf.lnk

Audio– use our calls as a resource to listen to any time

MP3 Version:
http://www.mediafire.com/file/gsxg0z72w1a095l/Get_Fit,_Lose_Fat,_Eat_Lots_Week_2.mp3

Links and Books

In Defense of Food by Michael Pollan
http://amzn.to/11fBXBf

Fiber http://www.hsph.harvard.edu/nutritionsource/fiber-full-story

Fiber, How Much?

http://www.webmd.com/food-recipes/features/fiber-how-much-do-you-need

Gatorade Nutrition

http://www.duetsblog.com/uploads/file/BairdGatoradeLabel.jpg

On to Week 3!

Chapter 8 Week 3

Settling In

"Have patience with all things, but chiefly have patience with yourself. Do not lose courage in considering your own imperfections, but instantly set about remedying the. Every day begin the task anew." – St. Francis de Sales

Words of Encouragement

The hardest part (getting started) is over and you have made it through the gate! Congratulations! Now let's move at a steady pace. For your sanity and success please remember to get out and sweat a bit 6 out of 7 days a week, even if only for 30 minutes.

Reminder: The Check List

Now is the time to revisit the official Check List, given to you last week! Have you:

__ Measured hips, thighs and waist?

__Taken a weekly photo?

__Checked your calendar and plugged in workout dates?

__ Shopped and prepared for the week?

__Allowed time to eat, savor a meal, eat with others?

__Taken supplements (if any)?

__Followed your activity and exercise routine?

Use this list weekly to check in on your goals and how things are coming along for you. Feel free to express questions or ah-ha moments, successes or challenges on the Facebook page – we'd love to hear from you!

Review of Last Week's Information

Last week we covered the importance of fiber, the amount of grams per day that is ideal to have in your diet and why grains and processed foods aren't supporting the work we are doing at this point in the program in relationship to blood sugar.

We reviewed the why and how regarding your exercise routine at a low intensity level, electrolytes and energy drinks, along with snacking to support exercise performance.

Topics Covered on This Week's Call

We add information regarding getting enough fiber - how to read carbohydrate and fiber ratios in the nutritional data on the back of some packages and also online through the links below that we have shared with you (under "Resources").

We delve further into questions regarding sodium and water intake, and the delicate balance our bodies need to maintain. Topics include hyponatremia (not enough salt intake); natural, mineral dense, colored salts and nutrients, how much is too much and when to add to cooking; pink, gray or Celtic sea salt flakes still have minerals intact, which helps keep the electrolytes balanced!

We begin to discuss moving ahead with eating and training after 6 weeks and what that looks like, touching briefly upon adding grains and more carbohydrates in different ratios. Yes, that's right! You get to eat grains again (eventually)!

Our Get Fit Facebook page is a great way to ask questions, express ah-ha moments and share recipe renditions. We spend a portion of this week's call answering your questions from Facebook. They include questions about:

1) Dairy and low fat milk

2) Keeping your heart rate at 65 – 70%

3) Lack of hunger, hard to eat first thing in the morning

4) Protein powders and meal supplements and which ones we recommend

5) More clarification on the 1:1 ratio

6) Creative recipe makeovers and how to dress up those greens or that chicken

Be sure to listen to the call to get the full download. For now, here are a couple of comments from past participants and their experiments with the recipes:

"I tried adding a little bacon to some collard greens and it was delicious!"

"My dinner last night… Chicken topped with gourmet mushrooms & sun-dried tomatoes. With roasted Brussels sprouts tossed with bacon, walnuts & dried cherries. Yum!"

A Bit More

Some of the best food out there is food you make yourself. Hopefully you have been venturing into your kitchen and trying out the recipes and menu options we have provided for you. Check out the handout outlining what makes up a whole foods pantry and what tools you might already have in the kitchen or might want to go grab and try out. Let us know if you love your lemon reamer or if your slow cooker is your favorite kitchen appliance!

Some Questions

1. What food combinations and recipes are you enjoying? How have you put your own stamp on them?

2. How does food taste to you? Are you finding you have to add more salt to your food, or are natural flavors more appealing?

3. Are any of your cravings going away or changing?

4. Have you posted or checked on the Facebook page yet?

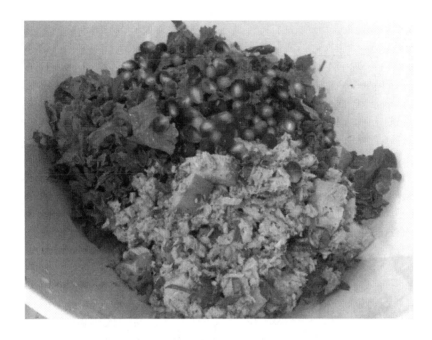

Salmon salad with pomegranate arils

Handouts, etc. from Week 3

Healthy Pantry and Kitchen Essentials

http://www.mediafire.com/file/hxyj7nwo080mje2/GET_FIT_
Healthy_Pantry_and_Kitchen_Essentials_handout.pdf

Menu Options #3

http://www.mediafire.com/file/f27cqxu6mb96i69/Week_3.M
enu_Plan_Additions.pdf

Audio – use our calls as a resource to listen to anytime

MP3 Version:

http://www.mediafire.com/file/emajocop40mjv5a/Get_Fit_Week_3_02012013.mp3

Recipe ideas:

Swiss Chard with Crisp Apples

http://blog.fatfreevegan.com/2013/01/swiss-chard-with-crisp-apples.html

Soup for a Healthy Cleanse or Just for the Great Taste!

http://www.refinery29.com/detox-soup?page=3

Food, food, and more food, the healthy kind

http://www.refinery29.com/food-bloggers/slideshow#slide-3

On to Week 4!

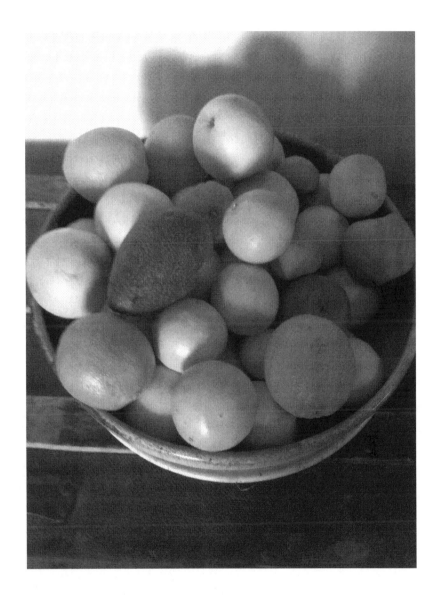

When you eat fruit, add protein to help control the sugar (and insulin) spike.

Chapter 9 Week 4

Seeing Progress

We want to congratulate you for the progress you've made over the past three weeks – you are running down the home stretch! And as we say weekly, tell us how you are feeling, give us some feedback and share with other participants how you are putting your own stamp on this program. Here is some feedback from past participants during Week 4:

1) Good energy and noticing the lack of irritable symptoms such as hot flashes – HUGE success

2) Weight loss

3) Inches lost – it's sinking in that muscle weighs more than fat

4) Meal planning is getting easier – just have to get used to it

5) Family meals and sneaking healthy food into the mix

6) Fun checking out the local food co-op, Whole Foods, natural food store or farmer's markets in neighborhood

7) Hormone and mood balancing

Fun family food includes garbanzo bean cupcakes, PB and J roll ups, chocolate hummus, avocado and chocolate pudding, veggies in tomato sauce. (You will find more suggestions linked at the end of this chapter and in your Menu Options handout).

The Checklist

Check back to your weekly list of action items from Week 2. This check list will remind you of all the progress you are making throughout the program.

A Review of the Last Week's Information

Last week we covered a bit more on the topic of fiber, focused on balancing sodium levels and the right kind of salt to add to your food, if any. We shared some feedback and answered questions that we received from our Facebook participants during the first program. We would love to hear from you, too, so join the Facebook group today and share your story.

Topics Covered on This Week's Call

Although fats have received a bad reputation for causing weight gain, fat is essential for survival. According to the Dietary Reference Intakes published by the USDA, 20% - 35% of calories should come from healthy fats. We need healthy fat, which we discuss in one of your handouts from Week 1 (Good Fat, Bad Fat) for:

1) Body to use vitamins

2) Brain development

3) Energy

4) Healthier skin

5) Healthy cells

6) Making hormones

7) Pleasure

8) Protective cushion for our organs

Healthy fats come from nuts and seeds, avocados, real butter, extra virgin olive oil and coconut. And the more pure the better; we recommend that you get natural peanut or almond butter without hydrogenated oils and preservatives. Read your nutrition labels and ingredients lists!

As we mentioned, most women need about 30% of their total daily calories to come from fat. For a woman eating 1,800 calories a day, that's around 540 calories from fat or 60 grams of fat each day, depending on your bio-individuality, of course. Here's what **60 grams of healthy fat might look like:**

- **1 Tbsp.** peanut/almond butter = 8 or 9 grams
- **1 Tbsp.** olive oil = 13.5 grams
- **1 ounce** almonds (around 23 almonds) = 14 grams
- **1/4 cup** sunflower seeds = 14 grams
- **4 ounces** cooked salmon = 14 grams

A Bit More

Thinking ahead, we start discussing eating and training, for the next phase, after six weeks, when you add in more carbohydrates in different ratios. For example, 30 to 60 minutes before your workout, make a smoothie with proportions of two or three parts carbohydrate to one part protein. Drink half pre-workout and half post-workout. Another option could be oatmeal, banana, hemp seeds, blueberries, nuts and low fat milk or yogurt. This will help to support more calories you burn as your training intensity increases.

This call will also cover additional Facebook posts, including:

1) Protein powder, benefits, costs and brands we prefer

2) Post-workout snacks include apple and nut butter, Larabar Uber Bars, homemade energy bars and roasted nuts. Exercise liquid snacks include coconut water, water or electrolyte replacement beverage…the possibilities are endless!

3) Meal suggestions for eating out

4) Using reasonable portions instead of exact measurements to achieve your 1:1 protein to carb ratio

Some Questions

1. What changes in your body, mood, energy or other physical markers have you found since getting started with us?

2. What is your favorite source of good fat? Love coconut in your smoothie, homemade guacamole or poached salmon with lemon and dill? Tell us on Facebook!

3. Have you heard of Michael Pollan? Check out his books online – easy reads, very informative and a great tool to assist you in your goals toward whole food health!

4. Are you checking your heart rate during and after exercise?

Handouts, etc. from Week 4

Healthy snacks for the whole family

http://www.healthykiddosnacks.com/1/post/2012/5/pb-and-fruit-rolls.html

Menu Options #4

http://www.mediafire.com/file/vc8v1qdmd4k7fqy/Week_4.Menu_Plan_Additions.pdf

*Audio – **use our calls as a resource to listen to anytime***

MP3 Version:

http://www.mediafire.com/?ypuow8jwww17521

Week 4 Reminder: *We call the program Get Fit, Lose Fat, Eat Lots because, as long as you act reasonably, you can **eat real amounts of real food**. No artificial, non-fat, tasteless, non-food items here! Your guideline is common sense and a food plan that will fill your nutritional needs along with a movement plan that will keep your physical body energized throughout the day.*

On to Week 5!

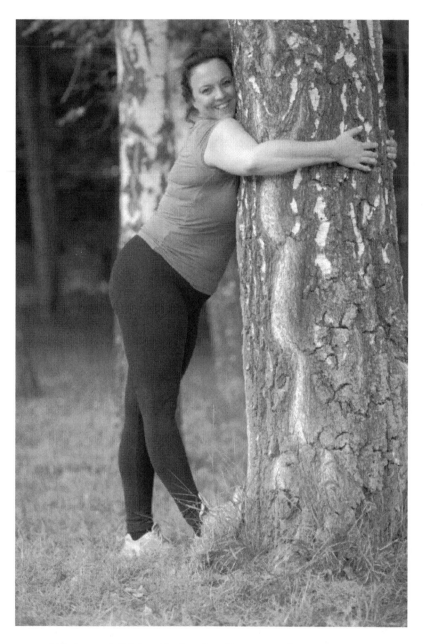

Life is good. Stick with the plan. You are making progress!

Chapter 10 Week 5

Almost There!

We are on the downhill run of our program, easing along the route with a bit more knowledge and awareness of how closely food and movement are tied together. We hope you are finding success with the knowledge and insight you have gained over the past few weeks...maybe even having some fun with it!?

The Checklist

Check back to your weekly list of action items from Week Two. This check list will remind you of all the progress you are making.

A Review of Last Week's Information

Last week we went over aiming to get 20% - 35% of your calories from healthy fats and how this is broken down. Additionally, we started discussing eating and training after six weeks, adding in more carbohydrates in different ratios and covered a few more Facebook inquiries.

Topics Covered in This Week's Call

Our bodies need balance. We are constantly moving along the path of maintaining homeostasis, literally balance within and without ourselves. It can be hard, we understand. But you are worth it! In Call 6, we discuss taking supplements in conjunction with eating whole foods, trying to get as many of your nutrients as you can from real food first. Check in with your primary care physician and/or your naturopathic doctor if you have specific questions.

As you know, keeping up with your physical training is critical throughout this program. We want to ensure you are getting at least thirty minutes of exercise at minimum, getting your heart rate up and sweating. The longer you exercise the better. Sweat it out!

Essential fatty acids are a great topic of interest when it comes to our health. They are essential in that our body cannot naturally produce these beneficial and crucial fats. We discuss how such foods as chia seeds, flax seeds and hemp seeds are great sources of omega 3 fatty acids, and we provide a delicious recipe for Banana Chia Pudding in your menu options handout for the week. Yum!

When incorporating grains back into the diet, you might come across information about soaking and sprouting grains. Wondering what the difference is and why you might want to do this? We discuss this in depth in our call and provide some links below on why and how this might be something to try in your household.

We will also focus on the topic of coconut milk versus coconut water and various nut and other "milks." Some people make their own nut and coconut milks because there are many additives found in commercial milks of this kind. We provide a recipe for you this week and challenge you to try out your own, to shift between homemade, when you have some extra time, and store bought when your time is limited.

A Bit More

If you eat a lot of food out of cans, you will find more information on BPA-lined cans and how they can affect your health in some of our links in Resources.

We continue the discussion about diet soda, and reiterate how soda can affect the body. There is suggestion for a proposed tax on certain portion sizes of soft drinks!

Some Questions

1. What supplements are you currently taking and why?

2. Do you drink dairy cow milk, goat milk, coconut milk, almond milk or something else? How do you use it in your diet?

3. What do you know about where your milk comes from? Is it local or from the other coast or what? Do you know what it means to be "ultra-pasteurized"?

4. What is your favorite way to use sprouted whole grain tortillas? With nut butter and banana, a little bit of chicken, cheese and lettuce, with some salsa? Do you cut some tortilla's up into wedges and bake them for homemade chips?

Handouts, etc. from Week 5

Menu Options #5

http://www.mediafire.com/file/exoz0zhi57srmiz/Week_5.Men u_Plan_Additions.pdf

Audio – use our calls as a resource to listen to anytime

MP3 Version:

http://www.mediafire.com/file/2bhtdb3h1duw29e/Get_Fit_W eek_5.mp3

Links

BPA and Cans - Are your canned goods safe to eat?

https://marksdailyapple.com/are-your-canned-foods-safe-to-eat-a-bpa-free-buying-guide

*Be Kind to your Grains **http://westonaprice.org/food-features/be-kind-to-your-grains***

BPA Free Version of Popular Foods/Mark's Daily Apple
http://marksdailyapple.com

Diet Soda Lies http://authoritynutrition.com/11-biggest-lies-of-mainstream-nutrition

Sprouting and Dehydrating

http://ournourishingroots.com/real-food-101-how-to-soak-sprout-and-dehydrate-nuts-benas-and-seeds

http://embracehn.com/holy-soaked-sprouted-and-dehydrated-buckwheat-batman/

On to Week 6!

Chapter 11 Week 6

Congratulations!

*With the first 10 days from Belly Fat Blowout 1 and this full 5 weeks in Book 2 you have completed the entire program called Get Fit, Lose Fat, Eat Lots – **Congratulations!** We hope some new habits have formed. Maybe new habits have replaced old habits that weren't serving you, or you found that you really, actually, truthfully do love to cook.*

As you continue on the path of eating and exercise and we will be available for basic guidance for your transition. Stay tuned for a book of recipes next along with a book for a more active lifestyle – increased activity and metabolic eating fit for an athlete in her different training phases.

Is a 5K race in your future? How about a 3 day breast cancer walk? A marathon? A hike through the Grand Canyon? Just more energy each and every day? There are so many activities to participate in when you feel good, eat well, and move on a regular basis.

The Checklist

As we end the program, remember to check back to your weekly list of action items from Week Two: measure your hips, waist and thighs, shop and prepare, etc. It is time to compare the progress you have made throughout the program. It might very well be time to go shopping for different clothes. We hope so!

A Review of Last Week's Information

We discussed taking supplements in conjunction with eating whole foods, keeping up with your physical training and why essential fatty acids are a topic of great interest when it comes to our health.

We reviewed incorporating grains back into the diet; touched on soaking and sprouting; mentioned different "milks" and how you can make your own; and read some controversial headlines on the topics of health and wellness.

Topics Covered on This Week's Call

We delve into myth busting and how to read and interpret articles with "loaded" headlines. Specifically, we focus on authoritynutrition.com "myth-busting" this statement, and our views on the topics "You should eat many small meals throughout the day."

Authority Nutrition states that, "The idea that you should eat many small meals throughout the day in order to "keep metabolism high" is a persistent myth that doesn't make any sense...It is true that eating raises your metabolism slightly while you're digesting the meal, but it's the total amount of food that determines the energy used, NOT the number of meals." We like some of the points made in this article, but this is how we begin to weigh in on our call:

1) It always depends on the individual! There are so many factors that matter here.

2) Exercise is essential! Carbs that aren't used for energy are stored as fat.

3) The article says "meals" not snacks

As you finish your first six weeks, you will be able to pick up the intensity of your exercise and will be eating a bit differently to accommodate this. We have started to outline the 2:1, carb to protein ratio. Be on the lookout for Book 3 as you transition into this next phase where grains enter again and a different ratio plays into what you eat as your activity increases.

A Bit More

We briefly discuss identifying hidden sugars and gluten in food, and the misconception that gluten free foods are healthier, have less calories and aren't refined. Check out the handouts provided for you this week for details.

Thank you for sharing this journey with us. It has been a pleasure working and growing together as we've progressed along the path of good health through exercise and whole foods eating. Remember the two go hand in hand: regular exercise and whole foods nutrition are wonderful and essential parts of life.

As always, we love hearing from you on our Facebook page! WE welcome your questions and feedback.

Eat well, continue moving, and be happy!

Handouts, etc. from Week 6

Recipe and Meal Options #6

http://www.mediafire.com/file/xp289x854ajb25s/Week_6.Me
nu_Plan_Additions.pdf

Audio – use our calls as a resource to listen to anytime

MP3 Version:
http://www.mediafire.com/file/zmrymctwkcpomg3/Get_Fit,_
Lose_Fat,_Eat_Lots_Week_6.mp3

Links

Should I Go Gluten Free?
http://www.mediafire.com/file/2523022p9thz8jo/Week_6_Gl
uten_Free_Handout.pdf

How to Spot Gluten or Hidden Sugar in Food
http://www.mediafire.com/file/3jzco89dh95cy31/Week_6_Ho
w_to_spot_gluten_or_sugar_hidden_in_your_food.pdf

Biographies

Stephanie Atwood M.A.

Best Selling Author, Award Winning Coach, Trainer, Sports Nutrition Consultant, and Ranked Masters Runner

When exercise and nutrition join forces there is a synergy that is almost like magic! When women of all ages, from 20 – 70 come together, for total health through fitness, friendship, and fun we call this Go WOW Team!

Stephanie Atwood is Bay Area Women's Fitness Writer, author of 3 Best Selling books on Amazon, and Founder of Go WOW Team, 2013 Winner Bay Area's Best Run Club. What sets her apart from the rest? She lives what she preaches and gets real results. Her dream is to bring fitness and overall good health to women, all ages, sizes, shapes and abilities.

Coach Stephanie offers women the opportunity to explore their own "athlete within" without judgment and with tremendous peer support. Until recently the missing component of the WOW Team Program was nutrition.

"We now incorporate a healthy approach to fat burning through the nutrition part of our program. Thus, when eating and exercise are combined, in an all-women's program, whole new worlds are opened for the women participating."

In Belly Fat Blowout and Belly Fat Blowout 2, Atwood and co-author Amy Griffith go into detail on how exercise and nutrition fit together. Through resources like the Get Fit Books, the WOW Team is growing into a national program with neighborhood workouts, online coaching, and printed materials.

Coach Stephanie's dream to bring women opportunity to rediscover optimal well-being, through food and movement, with support and encouragement, just keeps getting better every day! Go WOW Team and the Get Fit Book series are making this a reality.

Amy Griffith H.C. N.C.

First and foremost, I love food. As a certified Nutrition Consultant and Health Coach focusing on digestive distress, I assume my clients enjoy eating, too. I also empathize with them that it can be hard to tell the difference between what healthful food actually is and how they can get to a point where they are happy, healthy and satiated. This is the gap that I fill for my clients. Through my practice, Embrace Health & Nutrition, I provide people with customized health programs that fix the food first. I teach individuals how to prepare, cook and enjoy vibrant and delicious meals that mix flavor, color and nutrient density with a generous helping of love and mindfulness.

After working in the health care non-profit sector for nearly three years, I found my niche when I hired a nutritionist myself. I not only learned to love kale, but I learned who I was supposed to be: a personal nutritionist. My certifications as a Nutrition Consultant from Bauman College and a Health Coach from the Institute for Integrative Nutrition have equipped me with extensive knowledge in holistic nutrition, health coaching, and preventative health care. Drawing upon this knowledge of the science behind nutrition and the psychology behind how habits are formed, I work with clients to help them make changes that produce real and lasting results. I help my clients lift off the burden of having to make drastic changes and settle into a comforting, self-respecting lifestyle that promotes a higher quality of life.

I have had success with such health concerns as blood sugar regulation, pain management, food allergies and intolerances, digestive distress, weight loss/gain, autoimmune disease, nutrition for the athlete in training, and nutrition essentials for vegans or vegetarians.

In short, I believe that nutrition is the foundation that supports overall health and wellness, that quality of food is the key to enjoying, preparing and eating it, and that one size never fits all in regards to our bodies. This is the only life we have; we should give it our best.

Index to All Resources from this Book

If you would like a free copy of all of the links below in a PDF download please join our Live Fit Get Fit Mailing List and we will send it to you, absolutely FREE at http://eepurl.com/yLOWP along with a few other gifts.

Thank You!

Audio

1) **Week 1 Support Call**

http://www.mediafire.com/file/pp513bn1n1v8hx7/Get_Fit,_Lose_Fat,_Eat_Lots_Week_1.mp3

2) **Week 2 Support Call**

http://www.mediafire.com/file/gsxg0z72w1a095l/Get_Fit,_Lose_Fat,_Eat_Lots_Week_2.mp3

3) **Week 3 Support Call**

http://www.mediafire.com/file/emajocop40mjv5a/Get_Fit_Week_3_02012013.mp3

4) Week 4 Support Call

http://www.mediafire.com/?ypuow8jwww17521

5) Week 5 Support Call

***http://www.mediafire.com/file/2bhtdb3h1duw29e/Get_Fit_W
eek_5.mp3***

6) Week 6 Support Call

http://www.mediafire.com/file/zmrymctwkcpomg3/Get_Fit,_
Lose_Fat,_Eat_Lots_Week_6.mp3

Links, Etc.

BPA and Cans - Are your canned goods safe to eat?

https://marksdailyapple.com/are-your-canned-foods-safe-to-
eat-a-bpa-free-buying-guide

*Be Kind to your Grains **http://westonaprice.org/food-
features/be-kind-to-your-grains***

BPA Free Version of Popular Foods/Mark's Daily Apple
http://marksdailyapple.com

Diet Soda Lies http://authoritynutrition.com/11-biggest-lies-
of-mainstream-nutrition

Facebook Group Page
http://Facebook.com/GetFitSuccessTeam

Fiber http://www.hsph.harvard.edu/nutritionsource/fiber-full-
story

Fiber, How Much? http://www.webmd.com/food-recipes/features/fiber-how-much-do-you-need

Food, food, and more food, the healthy kind

http://www.refinery29.com/food-bloggers/slideshow#slide-3

Food Journal http://amzn.to/ZhmH3B

Gatorade Nutrition
http://www.duetsblog.com/uploads/file/BairdGatoradeLabel.jpg

Get Fit Cheat Sheet
http://www.mediafire.com/file/cffysesygd3f5f2/GET_FIT_Cheat_Sheet.docx

Good Fat Bad Fat
http://www.mediafire.com/file/wcfflz2eka78a1c/Good_vs_Bad_Fats_handout.pdf

Healthy Pantry and Kitchen Essentials

http://www.mediafire.com/file/hxyj7nwo080mje2/GET_FIT_Healthy_Pantry_and_Kitchen_Essentials_handout.pdf

Healthy Snacks for the Whole Family

http://www.healthykiddosnacks.com/1/post/2012/5/pb-and-fruit-rolls.html

How to Spot Gluten or Hidden Sugar in Food

http://www.mediafire.com/file/3jzco89dh95cy31/Week_6_How_to_spot_gluten_or_sugar_hidden_in_your_food.pdf

In Defense of Food by Michael Pollan
http://amzn.to/11fBXBf - *Book from Amazon*

Morning Mantras
http://www.mediafire.com/file/94k8qfv393dwe19/Embrace_
Health_Mantras.pdf

Recipes and Meal Options #1
http://www.mediafire.com/file/0ck7wk1mvml9e3a/GET_FIT
_Meal_Plan_WEEK_1.pdf

Recipes and Meal Options #2
http://www.mediafire.com/file/uzon9o32woeyntl/Get_Fit_We
ek_2_Menu_Options.pdf

Recipes and Meal Options #3

http://www.mediafire.com/file/f27cqxu6mb96i69/Week_3.M
enu_Plan_Additions.pdf

Recipes and Meal Options #4

http://www.mediafire.com/file/vc8v1qdmd4k7fqy/Week_4.M
enu_Plan_Additions.pdf

Recipes and Meal Options #5

http://www.mediafire.com/file/exoz0zhi57srmiz/Week_5.Men
u_Plan_Additions.pdf

Recipe and Meal Options #6

http://www.mediafire.com/file/xp289x854ajb25s/Week_6.Me
nu_Plan_Additions.pdf

Should I Go Gluten Free?

http://www.mediafire.com/file/2523022p9thz8jo/Week_6_Gluten_Free_Handout.pdf

Swiss Chard with Crisp Apples

http://blog.fatfreevegan.com/2013/01/swiss-chard-with-crisp-apples.html

Soup for a Healthy Cleanse or Just for the Great Taste!

http://www.refinery29.com/detox-soup?page=3

Sprouting and Dehydrating

http://ournourishingroots.com/real-food-101-how-to-soak-sprout-and-dehydrate-nuts-benas-and-seeds

Sprouting, More

http://embracehn.com/holy-soaked-sprouted-and-dehydrated-buckwheat-batman/

Sweat and Pulse/Heart Rate Information
http://www.mediafire.com/file/99m4j0nkaz2u8p0/Measuring_Sweat_and_Pulse_for_Healthy_Movement.pdf

Water!

http://www.mediafire.com/file/srgnvzt2lzr18zd/WATER.pdf.lnk

Weekly Food Prep Routine

http://www.mediafire.com/file/wry1t3muy5tkh1m/Weekly_Food_Prep_Routines.pdf

Your Ideal Day Timeline

http://www.mediafire.com/file/x4medodq5wdxa8p/GET_FIT_Your_Ideal_Day_timeline.pdf

Photo Credits

All photos not identified, were taken by the Authors or belong to the public domain

Cover Photo Credit - photos.com # 165424292

Photo #1 - Walking is a great way to move!

Photo #2 - Bacon and eggs starts a healthy breakfast

Photo #3 - Salad, wonderful, colorful, healthy salad

Photo #4 - Avocados are wonderful for you when eaten in moderation

Photo #5 - Nutrition facts/Kashi Cereal Label

Photo #6 - Shop the perimeter of the store! Better yet, start a garden!

Photo #7 - Working off the calories from sugary drinks - postgazette.com

Photo #8 - More nutrition facts

Photo #9 - A reasonable portion of chicken - http://www.webmd.com/food-recipes/nutrition-labels10/slideshow-serving-sizes

Photo #10 – Home-made soup

Photo #11 - Salmon salad with pomegranate arils

Photo #12 – Snack food

Photo #13 – Almost there! - photos.com # 15668194

*We call the program **Get Fit, Lose Fat, Eat Lots** because, as long as you act reasonably, you can **eat real amounts of real food**. No artificial, non-fat, tasteless, non-food items here! Your guideline is common sense and a food plan that will fill your nutritional needs along with a movement plan that will keep your physical body energized throughout the day.*

Join the Get Fit Family

Thank you for reading this book. Would you like to know when the next book is being published? Have a chance for a free book?

Join our mailing list at http://eepurl.com/yLOWP

If you enjoyed this book we would **love a review from you!** Here is the link to Amazon. It only takes 20 words. Thank you so much! http://amzn.to/19hyouV

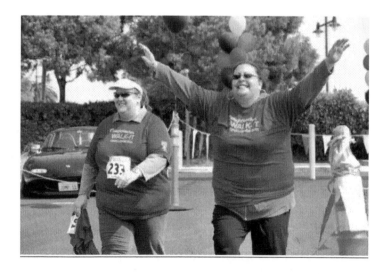

Happy, successful walkers from a Go WOW Team Walk-it 5K

Contact Us:

Stephanie Atwood at Go WOW Living

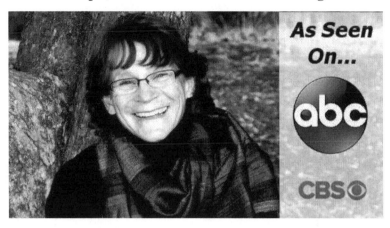

http://gowowliving.com or mailto:go@gowowliving.com

Go WOW Living on Facebook for National Women's Wellness Community

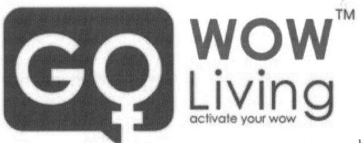

http:
//facebook.com/wowliving

Amy Griffith at Embrace Health Website

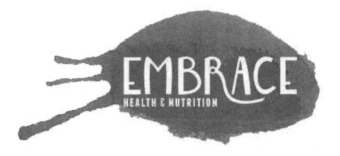

http://embracehn.com

Best Selling Books by Stephanie Atwood

Author Stephanie Atwood has written a number of books about health and fitness. Enclosed is a list with photos and a link to her author page showing all her books on Amazon.

Other books written by Stephanie Atwood

Belly Fat Blowout 2 http://www.amazon.com/Belly-Fat-Blow-out-Management-Moderate-ebook/dp/B00D0Y7EWU/

Freezer Meals – Comfort Food http://www.amazon.com/Freezer-Meals-Complete-Shopping-Convenience-ebook/dp/B00MRPKX58/

Freezer Meals Gluten Free http://www.amazon.com/Freezer-Meals-Shopping-Recipes-Convenience-ebook/dp/B00N7V76OM/

Run Faster Race Better http://www.amazon.com/Run-Faster-Race-Better-Triathlons-ebook/dp/B00BPIWJP0/

Run Faster Race Even Better http://www.amazon.com/Run-Faster-Race-Even-Better-ebook/dp/B00B8BRJYA/

Journal – A Day of Achievement and Inspiration http://www.amazon.com/Journal-Achievement-Inspiration-Stephanie-Atwood/dp/1494286149/

Leave us a review if you like what you read. Thank you again.

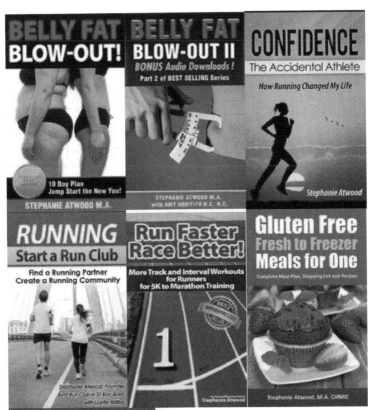

BELLY FAT BLOW-OUT!
10 Day Plan
Jump Start the New You!
STEPHANIE ATWOOD M.A.

BELLY FAT BLOW-OUT II
BONUS Audio Downloads !
Part 2 of BEST SELLING Series
STEPHANIE ATWOOD M.A.
with AMY GRIFFITH H.C. N.C.

CONFIDENCE
The Accidental Athlete
How Running Changed My Life
Stephanie Atwood

RUNNING
Start a Run Club
Find a Running Partner
Create a Running Community
Stephanie Atwood, Founder
Best Run Club in SF Bay Area
with Lizette NIÑO's

Run Faster Race Better!
More Track and Interval Workouts
for Runners
for 5K to Marathon Training
1
Stephanie Atwood

Gluten Free
Fresh to Freezer
Meals for One
Complete Meal Plan, Shopping List and Recipes
Stephanie Atwood, M.A. CHNRC

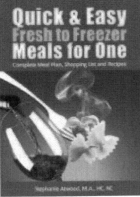

Quick & Easy
Fresh to Freezer
Meals for One
Complete Meal Plan, Shopping List and Recipes
Stephanie Atwood, M.A., HC, NC

Free Stuff!

Would you like to receive, **ABSOLUTELY FREE,** our e-publications **Top 10 Mistakes for Women New to Walking or Running** and **Good Fat, Bad Fat**?

Here is the link http://eepurl.com/xRm9L

Thank you and enjoy!

Disclaimer

This book is designed to provide helpful information on the subjects discussed. This book is not meant to be used, nor should it be used, to diagnose or treat any medical condition. For diagnosis or treatment of any medical problem, consult your own physician. The publisher and author are not responsible for any specific health or allergy needs that may require medical supervision and are not liable for any damages or negative consequences from any treatment, action, application or preparation, to any person reading or following the information in this book. References are provided for informational purposes only and do not constitute endorsement of any websites or other sources. Readers should be aware that the websites listed in this book may change.

This book is designed to provide information and motivation to readers. It is sold with the understanding that the publisher is not engaged to render any type of psychological, legal, or any other kind of professional advice. The content of any article is the sole expression and opinion of its author, and not necessarily that of the publisher. No warranties or guarantees are expressed or implied by the publisher's choice to include any of the content in this volume. Neither the publisher nor the individual author(s) shall be liable for any physical, psychological, emotional, financial, or commercial damages, including, but not limited to, special, incidental, consequential or other damages. Our views and rights are the same: You are responsible for your own choices, actions, and results.

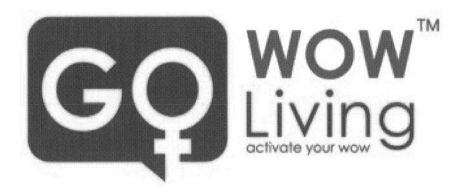

Please leave us a review on <u>Amazon.com</u> or other social media if you enjoyed these books.

Thank you!

<u>Back to the top</u>